What does LIVING WELL mean to you?

To me, **LIVING WELL** means doing everything I want to be able to do with the body and the mind God gave me. It means getting all the best resources and information I can find to make each day the best it can be.

LIVING WELL means that if I set a goal, nothing in my physical or mental world is going to be able to stop me. It means getting to a place where I can meet all the challenges of life.

LIVING WELL means going home at the end of the day and not feeling exhausted. It also means taking advantage of those opportunities to sit back and enjoy all the fruits of my hard labor.

I want to give you a prescription for **LIVING WELL** that comes from nature, not the drugstore.

I want you to live to at least ninety-eight healthy years old.

Until then I want you to be working, singing, dancing, Rollerblading, skateboarding, kickboxing, hiking, golfing, playing tennis, and chasing your spouse around the bedroom.

I want you to make love like a tiger.

I want you to prosper unbelievably at your job.

I want you to feel spiritually alive.

I want you to enjoy delicious food and regular fun and exercise with your family.

I want you to Live Well, look great, and feel spectacular, now and forever.

Together, let's make it happen—starting right now.

—from *LIVING WELL*

LIVING WELL

**21 Days
to Transform
Your Life,
Supercharge
Your Health,
and Feel
Spectacular**

MONTEL
WILLIAMS

WITH WILLIAM DOYLE

NAL

NEW
AMERICAN
LIBRARY

New American Library
Published by New American Library, a division of
Penguin Group (USA) Inc., 375 Hudson Street,
New York, New York 10014, USA
Penguin Group (Canada), 90 Eglinton Avenue East, Suite 700, Toronto,
Ontario M4P 2Y3, Canada (a division of Pearson Penguin Canada Inc.)
Penguin Books Ltd., 80 Strand, London WC2R oRL, England
Penguin Ireland, 25 St. Stephen's Green, Dublin 2,
Ireland (a division of Penguin Books Ltd.)
Penguin Group (Australia), 250 Camberwell Road, Camberwell, Victoria 3124,
Australia (a division of Pearson Australia Group Pty. Ltd.)
Penguin Books India Pvt. Ltd., 11 Community Centre, Panchsheel Park,
New Delhi - 110 017, India
Penguin Group (NZ), 67 Apollo Drive, Rosedale, North Shore 0632,
New Zealand (a division of Pearson New Zealand Ltd.)
Penguin Books (South Africa) (Pty.) Ltd., 24 Sturdee Avenue,
Rosebank, Johannesburg 2196, South Africa

Penguin Books Ltd., Registered Offices:
80 Strand, London WC2R oRL, England

Published by New American Library, a division of Penguin Group (USA) Inc. Previously published in a New American Library hardcover edition.

First New American Library Trade Paperback Printing, January 2009
10 9 8 7 6 5 4 3 2 1

The Traditional Mediterranean Healthy Diet Pyramid on page 126 provided courtesy Oldways www.Oldwayspt.org and www.MediterraneanMark.org.

 REGISTERED TRADEMARK—MARCA REGISTRADA

New American Library Trade Paperback ISBN: 978-0-451-22579-5

The Library of Congress has cataloged the hardcover edition of this title as follows:
Williams, Montel.
Living well: 21 days to transform your life, supercharge your health, and feel spectacular/Montel Williams with William Doyle.
    p. cm.
ISBN: 978-0-451-22293-0
    1. Nutrition—Popular works.   2. Exercise—Popular works.   3. Self-care, Health—Popular works.   I. Doyle, William, 1957–   II. Title.
RA784.W6385 2008
613.2—dc22   2007037799

Set in Scala and Univers
Designed by BTDNYC

Printed in the United States of America

PUBLISHER'S NOTE
Every effort has been made to ensure that the information contained in this book is complete and accurate. However, neither the publisher nor the author is engaged in rendering professional advice or services to the individual reader. The ideas, procedures, and suggestions contained in this book are not intended as a substitute for consulting with your physician. All matters regarding your health require medical supervision. Neither the author nor the publisher shall be liable or responsible for any loss or damage allegedly arising from any information or suggestion in this book. The opinions expressed in this book represent the personal views of the author and not of the publisher.
    The recipes contained in this book are to be followed exactly as written. The publisher is not responsible for your specific health or allergy needs that may require medical supervision. The publisher is not responsible for any adverse reactions to the recipes contained in this book.
    While the author has made every effort to provide accurate telephone numbers and Internet addresses at the time of publication, neither the publisher nor the author assumes any responsibility for errors, or for changes that occur after publication. Further, publisher does not have any control over and does not assume any responsibility for author or third-party Web sites or their content.

*This book is dedicated
to my family.*

A Note to the Reader

Contents

LIVING WELL

PART I: THE JOURNEY TO LIVING WELL

Introduction

The cameras are rolling.

I'm in my TV studio in New York, in the middle of taping an episode of my talk show.

I am listening closely to a guest on the stage, keeping my audience and production crew in the corner of my eye as my mind formulates a follow-up question.

I've been doing this for seventeen years. My competitors have thrown eighty contenders into the talk-show arena, and I've outlasted them all, every one of them. In fact, even after all these years, my ratings are up in key areas. I'm on top of the mountain, at the peak of my professional game.

The pain explodes inside of me without warning.

It feels like the earth has cracked open beneath my feet and flames are surging into my body, like someone's ramming a white-hot poker right up through the soles of my feet and jiggling it around inside my legs for a count of forty.

I am knocked practically off my feet. I teeter to keep my balance.

Barely hanging on until we call a commercial break, I stumble backstage and collapse into a chair.

For ten minutes, I sit there and weep.

Then I wipe my eyes, take a deep breath . . . and walk back onto that stage.

* * *

For the last eight years I've been living with multiple sclerosis, a potentially debilitating autoimmune disease that affects the brain and spinal cord.

One of the effects of my condition is that physical pain is a constant companion in my life.

The feeling ranges from a constant "dull roar" of pain that I feel all the time, 365 days a year—to episodes like this one that come close to hitting a ten on my personal Richter scale of pain, a feeling so intense that on two occasions I came very close to killing myself.

I am a fifty-one-year-old man who lives a very hectic life.

But I'm also living very well.

I've got a lot on my plate every day, lots of action and lots of stress. I'll bet you do, too.

I am a father and husband with a magnificent family. I am a CEO running three different businesses and about a hundred projects at a time, including writing this book. I'm an activist for health issues and patients' rights.

This week I'm traveling to four cities, speaking with twelve hundred to fourteen hundred people in each. Recently I was in eighteen different cities in two months.

Right now I'm in a hotel room in Los Angeles on business. Tomorrow I'm flying to Lansing, Michigan. Then I'll go back to New York for two days to tape new episodes of my TV program. Then I'll fly to Seattle, Washington, for two days. Then I'm off to Utah to recharge and go snowboarding for three days.

On my desk is a project list that runs on for several pages: review research for upcoming show tapings . . . check promo spots for the launch of my new *Living Well* DVD series . . . make notes for next annual meeting of the Montel Williams MS Foundation . . . review rundowns for appearances and meetings for the Partnership for Prescription Assistance . . . return over a hundred phone calls . . . etc.

Every single day, people walk up to me and ask me about my health. They stop me on the street and in airports, and say things like:

"Hey, Montel, I heard there was something wrong with you. But you look OK."

"Geez, Montel, you don't look sick. You look great!"

Sometimes that makes me feel good, and I appreciate people giving me positive thoughts. But sometimes it cuts very deeply and it almost hurts, because I am sick.

Just last week in my TV studio, a man in the audience stood up and said, "Montel, it's really funny, man. I heard a little while ago that you used to be sick or something? You used to have something wrong with you? But you look great, so everything must be good, right?"

My answer was "Thank you so much. I appreciate it. But believe me, I'm sick. You just can't see it, like you can't look around this room and pick out someone who has cancer. The truth of the matter is, you didn't watch me get out of bed this morning. Sometimes it takes me twenty minutes to get from my bed to the bathroom! Because ten minutes in between is me stuck on the chair crying because my feet hurt so bad."

I have multiple sclerosis, and that means I live with pain, and with limitations.

But the great news is that after consulting with the world's best experts and through intensive personal research and self-experimentation, I learned a truth that amazed me: *with the right diet and exercise, you can totally change your life for the better—no matter what your health is.*

That truly means that although I have MS, I can do things to ensure that it doesn't have me.

A couple of years ago, I began to intensify my search for ways to combat the symptoms of my illness.

Inspired by others who have successfully battled chronic diseases, I reviewed conventional and alternative therapies. I consulted the best scientific and medical experts around the world. I read piles of articles and research reports.

In the course of this journey of education and self-experimentation, I discovered a truth that completely transformed my life: *by supercharging your diet and physical fitness, you can reduce the risks and symptoms of chronic disease and vastly improve the way you feel.*

In my case, I learned that by pouring on the fruits and vegetables in their raw, fresh, whole, and blended forms; by slashing processed foods, junk foods, bad fats, and added sugars from my diet; and by following a special program of physical fitness, I could shrink the severity of my symptoms, rejuvenate my body and soul, and perform at a much higher level of intensity in all areas of my life.

Since I've been doing this, I can feel the difference in my bones—the bad days are further and further apart, the pain is less severe, and I feel better every single day.

Those earth-cracking-pain episodes I just told you about? They still happen periodically, but they are less frequent and more manageable. That makes a universe of difference to me.

And I've got some great news for you.

This style of Living Well is precisely what the world's best medical and scientific experts recommend to anyone interested in fighting chronic diseases like cancer, heart disease, obesity, and diabetes, and neurological diseases like MS—and for anyone interested in improving their overall health and longevity.

In this book, I'll show you how you can transform your life, fight disease, and feel spectacular.

I'll show you through my own stories, and an easy-to-follow 21-Day Living Well Program designed for superbusy people like you, with expert interviews, recipes, and workouts.

In this book, I will confess to you, move you, challenge you, provoke you, educate you, and inspire you to break through to a beautiful new level of Living Well.

I will give you the knowledge, the tools, and the motivation to transform your body, master your physical destiny, and feel spectacular.

Are you ready?

Let's do it!

CHAPTER 1

A Body Transformed: My Three Epiphanies on the Road to Living Well

Every morning of my life, I supercharge my body and soul.

I go to the refrigerator, take out a big glass bottle filled with a rich, beautiful green mixture, and pour it into a glass.

I bring the glass to my lips—and take a drink.

It feels like all the goodness of nature is flooding my senses.

It feels like my body is being drenched in a thick delicious haze of energy and power.

Instantly, I am awake, alive, sharp, and refreshed.

Within minutes, it kicks in fully and my whole body feels alive with energy and strength. My brain pops with ideas and plans for the day. I feel a sustained burst of energy that is almost beyond belief.

This Green Drink has become a crucial part of my life.

It helps explain the personal and professional victories I have in my life every day. It contains literally thousands of minerals, nutrients, and compounds that work together in an infinitely complex symphony of flavors and feelings and chemical interactions.

What's in the bottle?

It's a carefully blended mixture of the ultimate "superfoods": a rich variety of fresh organic fruits and vegetables, hand-selected for maximum taste and nutritional power. I rotate the ingredients: apples, oranges, carrots, spinach, mango, lettuce, kale, Swiss chard, beets, cantaloupe, bananas, asparagus, blueberries, strawberries, broccoli, collard greens, oranges, tomatoes, cabbage, and peaches.

Sometimes I'll blend in a small chunk of raw chocolate for extra sweetness. I blend in all kinds of fruits and vegetables, of every taste and color: from sweet to earthy to sour; and from purple, red, and orange to pink, blue, and electric green.

This Green Drink is my secret weapon. It's a power cocktail of nutrition. It gives me energy beyond belief. Why? Because it is brimming with some of the most beneficial substances in the nutritional universe: antioxidants, phytochemicals, fiber, flavonoids, polyphenols, and possibly a thousand other things we don't even know about yet.

And no matter who you are, whether you're perfectly healthy or if you're dealing with a health issue, these food compounds can help you reduce the risk of chronic disease and make you feel spectacular.

You absolutely need this stuff.

And you're going to love it!

Because it tastes like liquid heaven.

Believe me, I didn't always eat the healthiest food.

I was raised on a typical American diet from the 1960s that was heavy on things like meat, potatoes, white bread, and deep-fried chicken, and really light on fresh vegetables, fruits, and whole grains.

When I was growing up in Baltimore, we weren't exactly the richest family on the block. My parents were working as hard as they could to maintain our lower-middle-class status. They worked their tails off. My father sometimes worked three jobs, as a fireman, carpenter, and musician. I thought everyone's father had three jobs!

There were a few times when I was four and five years old and living in public housing that I remember eating nothing but pancakes for days. Eggs were really cheap back then, so we'd fill up on things like eggs and puffed rice to tide us over.

It's not like I was severely malnourished, but I was always a really skinny kid—rail thin. In junior high I looked emaciated: I was nearly six feet tall and weighed only 130 pounds.

When I entered the United States military and spent eighteen years on active duty, I ate some of the nastiest food on the planet. It was greasy, overcooked junk: the worst flour, the worst butter, the foulest federal cheese. I can't believe I survived this stuff!

Then I had three epiphanies over the years that changed my body and soul.

The first epiphany came when I accidentally became a hard-core bodybuilder.

I joined the armed forces upon graduation from high school, entering the United States Marine Corps first, then being accepted to the United States Naval Academy in Annapolis. While running one day, I snagged a curb with the side of my foot. I fell hard and ripped the meniscus in my left knee. By the time the surgery was finished, I went from running six to ten miles a day every day to a total standstill.

I was on crutches for nine months. My weight zoomed up from 147 to 182. To stay in some kind of shape, I started dragging myself to the gym every day and weight lifting.

I loved it. By the time I was in my twenties, I was lifting weights like a banshee. I was squatting 560 pounds on my back, bench-pressing 360, dead-lifting almost 600 pounds. I did this for a long time. My whole objective in life was to take up more real estate, boost my muscle mass, and cut my body fat.

If you spend lots of time in a gym, you'll hear every boneheaded nutritional theory and fad on earth: "Absolutely no carbs!" "More sugar!" "Less sugar!" "Protein, protein, protein!"

I chased after every fad, but I kicked them up to the extreme. I don't do things halfway—I try to push them to the stratosphere. I'm overpassionate about everything I do. I'm like the Energizer Bunny on rocket fuel.

I met a bodybuilder who told me that the best way to get your calories is to blend all your food, that grinding it up made your body bulk up more efficiently. So I would put a whole deboned chicken in a blender, add some tomato juice and potatoes, and blend the whole thing. How ridiculous is that?

Then I heard a guy in the gym declare that "grapefruit juice will burn fat." So every day for three months I downed about thirty ounces of crushed grapefruit juice! Is that good for you? I don't know!

Then another guy told me that if you mixed up a pile of powdered protein with orange juice and rainbow sherbet ice cream, you'd have so much sugar that it would "accelerate your metabolism" and help you "burn fat." So I'm telling you, for seven, eight months, I was guzzling that goop as my third meal of every day. What a fool.

I thought I would get healthy and strong this way.

But I was playing a silly game of trying fads based on no knowledge whatsoever. Ninety-nine percent of these theories were based on anecdotes, not any real science.

The good news that I had discovered bodybuilding, which has been a tremendously positive force in my life.

The bad news is that when it came to nutrition, I had no idea what I was doing.

My second epiphany happened one day in 1990, a few months before I started my talk show.

It was the day I realized I was eating garbage.

I was giving speeches to kids and young adults around the country about staying in school, staying off drugs, and making something of themselves. I spoke to 3 million kids across America, in more than a thousand high schools.

On this day I was at a high school in Gainesville, Texas. The gym teacher was escorting me around the campus on a tour before my speech. She was a gym teacher from central casting—attractive, six foot one, wearing a whistle around her neck and standard-issue blue sweatpants, yelling at people walking down the hallway.

We stopped into the cafeteria kitchen for lunch.

"What will you have, Montel?" asked the cook.

Now understand I had spent my whole life until then in a state of total opposition to vegetables, at least most of them. I'd tolerate mashed potatoes, fries, and the occasional green bean or tomato, but the sight of a salad or a Brussels sprout or a piece of spinach filled me with revulsion and contempt. I hated the sight of them. It was my personal war on vegetables. *You can keep your damn vegetables,* I'd think. *Don't let them come near me.*

"I'll have a piece of chicken," I told the cook, "and a piece of meat. That's all."

The gym teacher flashed me a look of surprise.

"Are you crazy?" she asked. "Is that all you're going to have? What about a vegetable?"

"I don't eat vegetables," I announced.

She bristled like I'd waved a red cape at her in the bull ring. "What are you talking about?"

"Well, they clog you up," I said. "They're bad for athletics."

Don't ask me where I got these dumb ideas from. I must have picked them up in the gym. If you'd asked me what my source was for these brilliant scientific theories, I'd have to tell you, "Hey, some guy told me!"

Well, that gym teacher laid into me for five minutes—and gave me an education I'll never forget. "You think you're going to talk to my kids looking the way you do? You look terrible! Your skin is paper thin. I can see every blood vessel in your body—that's not healthy! Look at you! You look borderline anemic!"

She was ripping me to pieces.

I had been traveling around the country for two weeks straight, eating exclusively in bad restaurants and junk-food joints. For breakfast, I was having eggs and grits, sausage and bacon. For lunch: chicken and French fries. Maybe a hamburger and a chocolate shake at night.

And I looked like crap, according to this lady.

She was just getting started. "How can you talk to kids and tell them to be healthy in mind and you're going to walk out there in a body that's not healthy?"

I stood in that kitchen completely dumbfounded. I didn't know what to say.

"Look at me," she said, pulling up her shirt to reveal a finely chiseled six-pack. "I don't lift weights, and I don't do half the exercise you do. But I'm eating healthy, living healthy, and my digestive system is running smoothly and efficiently. I would hate to look at your colon."

Hey, I thought, *I'd hate to look at anyone's colon.*

"Let's talk about this," she said, ushering me into her office.

Using flip charts and a book of government health guidelines, she gave me a crash course in the power of fruits and vegetables. The crux of the message was that I basically had little chance of living a healthy life without them. Lots of them, all the time, in many different shapes, types, and colors. I'd heard these things before, but never spoken about with such passion.

That woman woke me up like a slap in the face.

What if she's right? I thought. *Maybe I should start working this stuff into my diet.*

So I vowed, starting that day, every day, I was going to add really good things to my plate.

I started having a salad a day with dinner. Instead of eggs and bacon in the morning, I had eggs and a fruit cup. Eventually, I graduated to experimenting with green vegetables and gradually phasing more of them into my life.

And I was stunned to realize that they didn't taste that bad at all.

My third epiphany came years later, in 1999, when I was diagnosed with multiple sclerosis.

I was scared to death.

I'd heard of multiple sclerosis, but I didn't really know what it was. What I heard sounded like a death sentence. It meant excruciating pain and the possibility that I could eventually lose control of my body. This was enough to plunge me into the depths of despair.

In multiple sclerosis (the name means "multiple scars," which appear on the brain and the spinal cord), the immune system turns on and attacks the central nervous system, which can result in a whole lot of different symptoms. In my case, I suffer from severe tremors in my lower extremities, especially at night, plus extreme neuralgic pain in my feet, calves, and the back sides of my knees. There are days that the pain is so excruciating that I literally can't find my feet; I can't tell if my feet are on the floor or not. There were times it hurt so bad that I'd go into a closet and scream my lungs out. That pain helped plunge me into spirals of depression.

MS affects different people in different ways, and I don't want to trivialize or exaggerate other people's experiences. I'm just telling you what happened to me.

I also have balance problems, blurry vision, digestive problems, chest spasms, and trouble with swallowing. If you watch my talk show, you may have noticed that since I've been diagnosed with MS, I don't stand in the audience with my microphone asking people questions anymore; I have to sit on the stage. In bed, my legs twitch and shake like there's no tomorrow—I could bounce you right off the bed.

I'm usually feeling my best in the morning, so I try to work out and get as much work done as I can early in the day. But the simple act of walking is rarely easy. I have to think carefully about lifting up my feet, putting them down, and carrying on a conversation with someone at the same time. I'm thinking, *Lift right leg, walk, lift left leg, walk*, over and over all day.

When I stand up, I've got to hold on to something and think about the positioning of my legs. Otherwise I'd tumble right onto the floor. I have to get my brain to find my legs, take a test step, and find places to grab as I walk. Sometimes I even walk backward because I have more control that way.

Forget running; my brain just can't wrap itself around making my legs move, in that order, that quickly. If a fire breaks out in my room, I'm going to get out faster by dropping to my hands and knees and crawling out of the room. If somebody shoots a gun, I'm not going to run. I'm going to drop to the floor and crawl myself out of there.

Remember, this is just me. MS affects different people in different ways. But all of us with health challenges have a choice to make. We can sit back and just wait to see what happens, or take a proactive stand against the illness and in favor of our own health. I decided to take charge of my life, my health, and my medical care.

I read every book and article I could get my hands on, and I talked to countless people like myself who live every day with MS. I sought out the experts at Harvard Medical School and other top hospitals and universities. I traveled to Sweden for evaluation and treatment at the Karolinska Institute in Stockholm, which is the institute that presents the Nobel Prize in Medicine.

And I started searching for every edge I could find for feeling better and living well.

Then a friend of mine inspired me to push the idea of living well to a whole new level.

This woman looked terrific and exuded positive energy. Remember the line in *When Harry Met Sally*: "I'll have what she's having"? That's exactly what I thought when I met her.

She was very knowledgeable about fitness, food, and nutrition. I never saw anybody navigate their way around a restaurant menu with such authority. She wanted to know how food was prepared, what was in it, and if there were healthier choices available. To maximize her health and well-being, she wanted to put only the most nutritious food in her body.

Like that gym teacher in Texas, my friend believed that a key to living well was to get your digestive system working at its best by giving it the most healthful food you can find.

She cut refined and processed foods from her diet, and she favored olive oil over butter for cooking. And she was a huge fan of vegetables, especially raw vegetables. She stressed the importance of eating fiber- and nutrient-rich foods, especially for someone with a chronic health challenge like me.

I thought I was eating pretty healthy already, but she was pushing the idea even further, and I was intrigued.

I am intellectually very curious, and I open my mind to all approaches to health: conventional medicine, nontraditional and alternative therapies, acupuncture and Eastern medicine.

When it comes to health and fitness, I am simultaneously very open-minded and very skeptical. As Dr. Andrew Weil once said: "I am open to lots of things. Then I want to see the proof."

One day my friend brought me a freshly blended green vegetable drink from a health-food store. "Try this," she said. It looked like a glass of green paint—in fact, it looked downright nasty—but I braced myself and drank it down.

It tasted funky, but as I chugged it down, the strangest thing happened. It gave me a burst of energy so strong, I swear I could feel the nutritional power of the drink flood through my body.

It blew my mind!

I started knocking down two green drinks a day. One of the things that really frustrated me about MS was the digestive problems it caused; sometimes I just couldn't get my bowels moving for two or three days, because the natural peristalsis motion inside my stomach was too weakened. By the third or fourth day of green drinks I noticed a change in my bathroom habits. I started going to the bathroom once, then twice a day. I started feeling better and better.

After three months of this, I realized I could whip up my own Green Drinks at home, and I could make them taste way better than the health-food store's. So I bought a Vita-Mix machine and started blending my own juice drinks and smoothies at home every day, experimenting with different fruits and vegetables.

I started feeling wonderful. My MS symptoms started getting less severe. I felt lighter on my feet. I felt less pain.

The positive impact of the Green Drinks inspired me to go even further.

What would happen, I thought, *if I pushed the idea of healthy eating as far as I could? How far could I go, and how good would I feel?*

I pulled most of the white flour, sugar, and table salt out of my diet and switched to whole-grain breads and cereals. I started eating twenty salads a week. I not only radically improved the quality of what I was taking in, I "switched out" a lot of the less healthy stuff—no red meat, no chicken, no pizza, no junk food.

And then I fell in love with raw foods.

I already told you how carried away I can get. I went almost 100 percent raw, focusing on lots of fruits and vegetables and the occasional piece of cooked fish.

Working with a raw foods chef, I based my diet mainly on raw, whole fruits and vegetables, green juice drinks, blended fruit and vegetable smoothies, protein smoothies, and raw soups.

I had lasagna made of cucumbers and squashes and nut milk and nut cheese. I'd take an entire chopped salad, throw it in a Vita-Mix, grind it all down, and eat it as a soup, cold. I'd take an orange, a mango, a whole head of lettuce, and a whole head of spinach, grind it up in the blender and guzzle it down, all the pulp and everything.

I did this for ten months straight—raw and whole foods, juice drinks and smoothies every day.

And let me tell you, everything about me and my illness got better.

My body felt significantly improved, with less pain from day to day. My average "walking-around pain" used to be roughly 5 out of 10, with 10 being the worst, where it cracked my core and I was ready to kill my-self. But now it only averages around a 3.5.

Previously, I had been on various antidepressant medicines to cope with the depressive episodes that my physical pain made worse. This new eating regimen helped my depression, without a doubt. I felt that my ebbs and flows were softer, that the emotional swings were not as severe, and I didn't go into such deep spirals of depression. I felt the need for less medicine. The bad feelings were further and further apart.

But with diets, as with anything, I think you can go too far, especially when there isn't good medical or scientific evidence to back them up.

Just look at all the information floating around on the Internet, in health-food stores, and elsewhere about detoxing and jump starts and colon cleanses. Some of these regimens are so extreme and dangerous that they may harm the body. I've met people who have done these four- or five-day "cleanses" and they look to me like they're getting sick and don't even know it.

A while ago, I met a raw foods chef who never touched any animal flesh, ever. I don't want to put the guy down, but he looked like a weak thirteen-year-old girl. His bones were about as big around as my finger and his skin looked waxy.

The main problem for me when I went almost 100 percent raw was that I lost so much weight. I went from 196 pounds to 179 in just seven weeks. A friend pulled me aside and said, "Montel, you're getting too thin!" Even though this is well within the normal healthy weight range for my body type, I was a six-foot-tall man with a twenty-nine-inch waist, which is kind of ridiculous.

So I did my homework and tracked down the best research and expert opinion I could find. And I learned that not everything in the "raw foodist" gospel is necessarily true. One recent study even suggested that if you go too far to an extreme in pursuing a raw foods–only diet, you can actually increase your risk factors for heart disease. Going to radical extremes is rarely a good idea when it comes to your health.

Raw foodists are sometimes right for the wrong reasons: leafy greens *are* extremely healthful, not because they are more "alkaline," but because like most fruits and vegetables, they are rich in nutrients and fiber, and they help you feel fuller more efficiently than things like fast food.

Raw foodists believe that cooking vegetables destroys plant enzymes that the body needs in order to absorb food nutrients. But nutritional experts dismiss this claim. Some raw foodists believe that sea salt is better for you than regular salt. But it turns out that there's really no significant nutritional difference between them.

What most experts agree on is that a plant-based diet rich in vegetables and fruit is fantastic for your overall health, and you can enjoy produce in a variety of different forms and cooking styles: raw, fresh, canned, frozen, cooked, or steamed.

So now I strike more of a balance in ultra-healthy eating. I enjoy raw food—and I enjoy cooked food. I've added some more fish back into my diet. I've added some meat back into my diet. I'll sometimes have a sandwich, preferably on whole-grain bread. I've even enjoyed some cookies and the occasional pizza. Comfort food is good for you now and then!

Some people follow an absolute "100 percent raw" diet. If it works for them, and their doctors say it's OK, then that's great, and I say more power to them. But I don't need to be 100 percent raw. I'm fifty-one years old; I've been enjoying all kinds of food for most of my life. I've been an athlete my whole life, and I've been eating meat my whole life. I can't just wean myself totally off it and say "no more meat—forever!"

Now I eat a piece of steak every five or six days. I'll have a really nice cut of meat, like a T-Bone, or a piece of sirloin or rib eye or New York strip on the bone.

That steak is good for me! It helps me maintain my muscle mass, my body weight, and my brute-strength endurance. That comes, in part, from having the protein and iron from that meat. For me to be able to lift the weights I lift, I need some meat. When I'm on a 100 percent "all-green" diet, I'm not as strong. So I obviously need it. I just don't have to eat steak every day.

For breakfast yesterday I had two egg whites and one yolk, a little cheese, and a bowl of strawberries. Lunch was a nice piece of salmon with some miso glaze. Dinner was a mouthwatering pulpy soup made from six different raw vegetables. Tonight, I'll have a big salad and some fish. Tomorrow I might go out and have a burger, or some really good hormone-free Kobe beef, with beets and spinach on the side.

On top of this, every day I enjoy a nutritional triple play of a Green Vegetable Drink in the morning, a Sweet Green Vegetable-and-Fruit Smoothie at midday, and a Fruit Smoothie in the afternoon, all of them made from fresh, whole, raw produce. This way, I wind up consuming an average of four or five medium-sized healthy meals every day.

I feel fantastic. Plus, I'm staying consistently around 185 pounds, which is close to an ideal weight for me.

What does Living Well mean to you?

To me, Living Well means doing everything I want to be able to do with the body and the mind God gave me. It means getting all the best resources and information I can find to make each day the best it can be.

When I was first diagnosed with MS, the doctor basically told me, "You need to go home and try your best to prepare to die."

Instead, I decided to go home and prepare myself to live every second of my life to its 100 percent fullest. Period.

I could sit back and say, "MS really has me." But instead, I decided *I* have *it*. It doesn't define me, and I will not let it define me. What will define me is all those incredible, positive things I can do for myself in my everyday life.

Every day, I'm going into battle to achieve victory in my personal and professional life, and every day I'm going to battle against an illness. I believe you've got to have everything you can possibly have in your arsenal if you're going into battle.

Living Well means that if I set a goal, nothing in my physical or mental world is going to be able to stop me. It means getting my body and my mind to a place where I can meet all the challenges of life that I put before me: my family, my work, my ambition, and the goals that I've set.

Living Well means going home at the end of the day and not feeling exhausted. I want to go home feeling good, like I've put in a good day's work, and now I'm going to get some rest so I can get up and do it again tomorrow.

But Living Well also means taking advantage of all those opportunities I have to sit back and smell the roses and enjoy all the fruits of my hard labor. Every now and then you've just got to take some time to rest, to relax, to enjoy.

Living Well means that when I get up in the morning, if I feel like playing basketball, or scootering with my kids, or going out and jumping up and down in the ocean with my family, I'll be able to do it and not run out of gas in the first few minutes.

Every night before I go to sleep, I ask myself the same question: "What did I do today that's worth talking about tomorrow?" I look for every opportunity to just do something different today, something good today. As I end every single day, I never close my eyes without asking myself that question. It helps me end my day proud, and starts my next day with a success.

In the morning, I have these weird little conversations with myself, all alone in the bathroom, hands on the counter, looking in the mirror.

Those eyes that are looking back at me don't lie. They'll tell me,

"Damn it, my body hurts." So I'll say, "Well, what are you going to do about it? Get your ass up and go to work, Montel—*Go!* You did it yesterday, and you can do it today!"

Then I immediately go into the kitchen and grab a Green Drink. It's something positive I can do for my body that will make me feel good.

I'm standing on top of a nine-thousand-foot mountain on a crystal-clear blue-sky Utah morning, ready to pounce into space. Scattered hawks are drifting in lazy circles over pine trees in the vast canyons below.

My feet are strapped into a five-and-a-half-foot-long fiberglass snowboard. My iPod is locked and loaded with Dr. Dre, Frank Zappa, Snoop Dogg, Anastasia, Grover Washington, Jr., and Christina Aguilera. I look like a gladiator: I'm wearing motocross upper-body armor, a steel crash helmet, goggles, leather wrist guards, and ballistic padding on my shoulders, butt, knees, and back. I've got two-way radios and a GPS in my pocket.

I inhale a blast of cold air, crank up the music, and push off.

I know those mountains like the back of my hand, and soon I'm riding hard, leaning into the slope and cutting winding turns into the smooth, fresh powder. I go faster and faster, bouncing from side to side, hitting forty-five miles an hour as I skip around a patch of trees, spot a bump on the trail, and shoot it into the air.

All my life I've been an exercise hound, and my regular workout regimen includes lifting weights, riding stationary bikes that also exercise the arms and trunk, swimming in a pool, running, and practicing martial arts. And today I'm enjoying the most outrageously enjoyable exercise I've ever dreamed of.

Something almost miraculous happens to my body when I snowboard. I'm a middle-aged man who's had a debilitating neurological condition for seven years—but today I feel like an Olympic athlete in peak condition.

Usually, the simple act of walking is a pretty complex task for me. But now I am completely transformed. The signals between my brain and limbs are razor-sharp. Everything is working together like a symphony:

feet, ankles, calves, thighs, hips, eyes, and upper body. Snowboarding has been a godsend for me, and I think it may help my brain's ability to process where the body is in space.

After a day of snowboarding, I'll walk better than I have in weeks. It's like night and day for my balance and walking. The benefits last for days. Without a doubt, snowboarding has helped my MS.

And it's amazing how good I have been feeling.

I've always said that in this country we look at illness as weakness. Well, I may be ill, but I'm for damn sure not weak! And I'm not going to let myself be weak. If my body plays tricks on me, then I'll be as strong as I can be in whatever body I have.

I've been able to mitigate some of the symptoms that I have, or at least lessen their severity. I am convinced that my diet and physical fitness have helped prevent MS from ravaging my body the way it could have. I think the more I stay with this, the better and better I'll be.

I've learned three major physical lessons for Living Well:

- **Living Well Lesson #1:** I sharply boosted the amount and variety of fruits and vegetables in my diet, especially their raw, fresh, whole, juiced, and blended forms.
- **Living Well Lesson #2:** I exercise regularly at a moderate-to-high level of intensity up to sixty minutes a day, on most days of the week.
- **Living Well Lesson #3:** I gradually switched out processed and refined foods, junk foods, bad fats, and added sugars from my diet—and switched in good fats from sources like fish and good carbohydrates from whole grains.

The result is that I've transformed my body and rejuvenated my spirit, and I now perform at a much higher level of intensity in all areas of my life.

These lessons helped me achieve a heightened new awareness of Living Well and living life to its absolute fullest.

And right now a rising chorus of the most distinguished doctors, scientists, and medical researchers around the world is telling you and me that these lessons are a key not only to Living Well but to living longer and healthier, and fighting chronic diseases like obesity, diabetes, cardiovascular disease, and several forms of cancer.

You can do this, too, and I believe it can totally change your life for the better.

Of all the things I've done in my professional life, there's one project that I may be the proudest of. For the past year, I've been the national spokesperson for the Partnership for Prescription Assistance (PPA), a huge campaign by the pharmaceutical industry to get prescription drug help to all Americans who need it.

My face has prompted over 12 million people to call the PPA's phone number. There has never been a private-sector initiative in American history where business has given away more of its product: in this case, $10 billion.

That's 10 billion dollars' worth of medicine given away directly to people in need—because of my mug—my face. Robin Hood's got nothing on me!

We can criticize the pharmaceutical industry and Western medicine all we want, and sometimes quite rightly, but sometimes we really need them. In fact, one of those medicines is the reason I'm alive today.

But what is truly mind-blowing to me is that tens of millions of Americans are taking medicines for chronic diseases that are worsened or even caused by unhealthy diets and a lack of exercise. In other words, they are largely self-inflicted diseases. How tragic is that!

Right now there are multitudes of our brothers and sisters across the United States in hospital beds and intensive care units, their limbs amputated and hearts failing, suffering terribly and dying, all because of the cumulative damage of years of unhealthy diets and sedentary lifestyles.

This is outrageous! It shouldn't be happening!

These people should have had the tools, the knowledge, the resources, and the motivation to be proactive in Living Well through prevention.

I wrote this book to help you start paying attention to your diet, your exercise, and your health *right now*, before you have to go to the doctor and get a prescription filled.

I want to give you a prescription for Living Well that you can get from nature, not the drugstore.

Living Well is a four-legged stool: spiritual, emotional, financial, and physical. This book is about Living Well physically, which in my opinion greatly influences the other three legs.

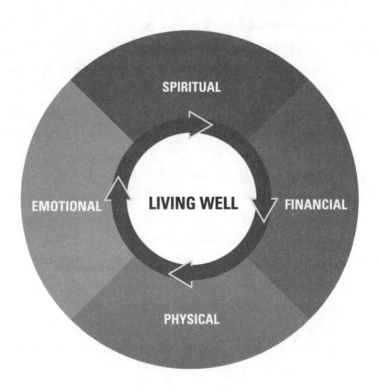

To help us in our journey, I reached out to a very distinguished "dream team" of some of the greatest scientists, doctors, and university researchers in the United States for their opinions for this book.

I picked their brains, reviewed their latest research, and asked them a series of questions on one major theme—how can you and I Live Well?

I want you to live to at least ninety-eight healthy years old.

Until then, I want you to be working, singing, dancing, Rollerblading, skateboarding, kickboxing, hiking, golfing, playing tennis, and chasing your spouse around the bedroom.

I want you to make love like a tiger.

I want you to prosper unbelievably well at your job.

I want you to feel spiritually alive and I want you to amass a multimillion-dollar fortune if you want to.

I want you to enjoy delicious food and regular fun and exercise with your family.

I want you to Live Well, look great, and feel spectacular, now and forever.

Together, let's make it happen—starting right now.

The Dream of Living Well

I **recently met an amazing American family.**

They are the Quance family: mom Melissa, dad Dale, and their four children.

Like a lot of Americans, they have a weight problem.

What's remarkable about the Quances is that they were so concerned about their weight and their health that they came on my show to talk about it before a national TV audience. In my book, that takes some guts.

Melissa told me frankly, "I have been overweight for the last thirteen years." One of her goals in life was simply to feel good in lingerie. She worried that her kids were being picked on because they're overweight, and she worried that they might eventually get heart attacks.

Dale is a soda-and-chocolate-loving guy who had also been over-weight for years and wished he had more energy. Daughter Brittany was barely into her teens and she already weighed 160 pounds. How did this happen? Brittany put her finger right on the heart of their predicament: "The problem in this family is what you eat, and how much of it you eat." They simply ate too much bad stuff, all the time. Her younger sister Ash-leigh explained, "If I want junk food, nobody can stop me."

"We are a family that lives in the fast lane," said Melissa, "so the fast food is the way we go." Sometimes they ate fast food seven times a week. "We buy pop, chips, ice cream, frozen pizzas, chicken nuggets, brownies, cookies," confessed Melissa. "When we snack, it's chips and cheese."

Does this maybe sound a bit like your family?

The Quance family really wanted to change their lives for the better.

They wanted to Live Well, be healthy, and feel great. They asked for my help, and I was happy to give it.

So I asked my Living Well coach Chris Freytag to come into their home and give them a crash course in healthy living. Chris is a health and fitness coach, and is also *Prevention* magazine's fitness expert and contributing editor. She is a powerhouse of positive energy and knowledge.

As the family looked on nervously, Chris pulled open their refrigerator and looked inside. It was a full-blown nutritional hell zone. It was not unlike many American family kitchens, but Chris was still shocked by what she saw. Bologna. Jumbo hot dogs. Sugared soda. Stacks of frozen pizzas. All kinds of processed foods. "What are you having for breakfast over there?" Chris asked Brittany. The reply: "Pizza." Can you believe it, pizza for breakfast!

"The very first thing we've got to do," announced Chris, "is dump the junk." Then she cleaned out that whole kitchen. All the junk went into the garbage. "Oh, no," protested Ashleigh, "not my cookies!" Out they went.

Next, Chris took them to a Whole Foods supermarket for a lesson in shopping healthy and shopping smart. Then she put together a workout they would do in their house, all together as a family: squats, stretches, some cardio, lots of huffing and puffing. Finally, they came on my show to tell me their story.

I was so impressed by the Quances' determination to make their lives better. I looked into their faces and I could tell they were so sick of being overweight, and they were hopeful and excited about getting healthy. But I told them they've got to make real changes and stick to them.

What's the Quance family's biggest problem? Time, they told me. They're always in a hurry, always rushing. Their lives are so busy they can't find the time to eat healthy or exercise. Sound familiar?

I told them, "You guys need to sit down and take a big calendar of the week and put the schedule up on a board and ask yourself, 'What are we wasting time doing?' Because if you don't have enough time to go shopping and actually stop to look at what you put in your body, everything else you're doing is a waste of time. I'm sorry. I've got to say it. The most important thing you can do in your life is what goes in your body."

I believe this with all my heart, and I want you to believe it, too: *it all starts with what you put into your body*. If we don't get this right, we won't perform at our peak in life, in love, with our families and our careers. You've simply got to get this right first.

I believe this is doubly important for anyone facing a health challenge, like I am, whether it is heart trouble, arthritis, neurological disease, cancer, or simple overweight.

You've got to have a body that's functioning at its best level, based on what's going into it, and not stressed out from having to digest all the chemicals, extra garbage, and pure waste material in processed food. That body will be better equipped to deal with the challenges it faces.

It's no secret that eating well and exercising make you look better, makes you feel better, and makes you healthier.

But a lot of people think that making a change would be way too difficult. The reality is it's pretty simple, probably much simpler than you think. And the simplest changes can make the biggest differences in your life.

People write to me all the time and say, "Montel, how do you stay in shape?" "How do you look so good?" "What's your secret?" Well, I stay on top of my diet, I stay on top of my medication, I stay on top of every aspect of my life, and I exercise.

I also try my best to focus on my mental health, because one of the top side effects of this disease is depression, so I work very, very hard at it every day to make sure that I stay in control as best I can.

But it all begins with what you put into your body. That's really the ticket for getting yourself on track to a good, positive, healthy life. We have to make better choices in what we eat.

Unfortunately, millions of Americans are headed in exactly the opposite direction. This is the story we hear from across the country, from mothers, fathers, schools, and everybody: we have an entire generation now that is making bad choices.

Far too many of us are getting fatter, sicker, and more physically miserable every day. And it really hurts. I met a woman on my show named Tammy who weighed 320 pounds at age thirty-eight. She just wanted to be able to run around and play ball with her kids, and to have her husband hold her and be able to fit his arms around her. She wanted so badly to lose weight. "I'm not sure how I'm going to do it," she told me, "but someday I want to look at myself in the mirror and say, 'I love you, Tammy,' and really believe it."

Don't get me wrong: I'm all in favor of people getting fit at any weight. We still have way too many dangerously skinny models in our pop culture, and they're setting a lousy example for our kids. I think that full-figured people possess just as much authentic human beauty as anyone else, and I hate how overweight people, especially kids, can be teased, ridiculed, and shamed.

I had on my show a young woman named Ashley who was a high school cheerleader, but was teased relentlessly about her weight. "Kids would call me a horse," she said. "They'd put horse feed in my locker at school. They would neigh at me as I walked past them. And it finally got so bad that a girl made posters of a horse's body and put my head on it, and passed them all over." Eventually she was forced to change schools.

That makes me furious. It makes me crazy. How dare anyone make fun of a person because of their weight!

THE BAD NEWS: OUR DIETS ARE HIGHLY DANGEROUS

The trouble, however, is that beyond their impact on our self-esteem and emotional well-being, overweight and obesity are very real health threats to our kids and to all of us. They can hurt you—and they can literally kill you.

What are the health risks of obesity? According to the World Health Organization, obesity is associated with:

- premature death
- heart disease and stroke
- damaging effects on blood pressure, cholesterol, triglycerides, and insulin resistance
- type 2 diabetes (high blood sugar)
- cancers, including breast, colon, prostate, endometrial, kidney, and gallbladder
- sleep apnea (when breathing is interrupted during sleep)
- osteoarthritis (wearing away of the joints)
- gallbladder disease
- irregular periods
- problems with pregnancy, such as high blood pressure or increased risk for cesarean section (C-section)
- respiratory difficulties, chronic musculoskeletal problems, skin problems, and infertility

That's one hell of a list, isn't it?

Don't forget that diabetes, for example, is not just a medical term; it is a slow-motion, flesh-and-blood horror movie that can result in all kinds of physical disasters in your body, including blindness, kidney failure, impotence, infections, and the amputation of arms and legs.

And right now things are getting so bad in our country that for the first time ever, our children are being routinely diagnosed with high blood pressure and *adult-onset* type 2 diabetes! The number of overweight children has doubled and the number of overweight adolescents has tripled since 1980.

Last year, *People* magazine reported on a girl in Arkansas who ate a diet of Froot Loops, Frosted Flakes, pizza, Wendy's, McDonald's, Popeye's, and Red Lobster crab legs with butter. She was just a six-year-old girl, and already she weighed 120 pounds and suffered from high blood pressure!

We are turning our kids into train wrecks—and ticking time bombs. "Obesity is the terror within," announced U.S. Surgeon General Richard Carmona in early 2006. "Unless we do something about it, the magnitude of the dilemma will dwarf 9/11 or any other terrorist attempt."

Incredibly, Surgeon General Carmona described obesity as a national security crisis for the United States, asking, "Where will our soldiers and sailors and airmen come from? Where will our policemen and firemen come from if the youngsters today are on a trajectory that says they will be obese, laden with cardiovascular disease, increased cancers and a host of other diseases when they reach adulthood?"

We are becoming the fattest people on this planet. This country is overeating, miseating, and couch-potatoing itself right into the hospital, into intensive care, and into early graves. Two-thirds of Americans are overweight or obese.

MORE BAD NEWS: OUR LIFESTYLES ARE SABOTAGING OUR HEALTH

Why are so many Americans out of shape?

What happened to us?

There are dozens of reasons—we've got bigger portions, more junk food, more hectic schedules, and more sedentary-inducing technologies, like e-mail and video games.

But in a larger sense, we've allowed our lifestyles to overwhelm our priorities. Here's a typical day in the life of many Americans:

I'm late. Skip breakfast. Rush out the door, race to the car; get to the office early enough so I can check my e-mails in case my boss asks me about something that happened.

Go to a meeting in the conference room; grab one of those sticky hockey-puck pastries with a mysterious glop of simulated fruit in the middle.

Sit at my desk all day looking out of the corner of my eye at my computer screen to watch the news and incoming e-mail.

Scarf down a fast-food lunch at my desk. Get full fast. Get sleepy.

Slurp down a triple-whipped iced coffee-chocka-chino with extra foam, perk up, write ten memos.

Instead of walking twenty feet down the hall to pop my head into a colleague's office, send her an e-mail. Faster. More efficient. I don't have to move a muscle.

Get off work; switch on the BlackBerry while I drive so I can see if my boss needs something.

Pick up sodium-and-saturated-fat-drenched "curbside takeaway" dinner from the family restaurant next to the mall. Call ahead and they pass the bags right through my car window so I don't even have to stand up.

Go home, wolf down dinner and pie from plastic containers, collapse in exhaustion on the floor like a root vegetable. Worship the plasma TV gods for three hours. Suffer from electronic stupor and eyestrain.

Sleep, wake up, do it all over again, like a frantic mouse in a spinning wheel.

How crazy are we? We used to joke about the downfall of mankind, and look at what we've become! It's already happening. We're all in there spinning around on that hamster wheel, trying our best every now and then to look to the right and the left to see if we're doing better than our neighbors and to prepare for the next thing we have to do. Only we're not really spinning—we're sitting on our butts much of the time.

The United States is a gigantic booby trap of unhealthy lifestyles and bad nutrition. We're spending much of our lives in our cars eating fast food. The typical American diet is abysmally low in fruits, vegetables, and whole grains, and much too high in calories, sugar, salt, and saturated fat. As a result, tens of millions of us are obese or overweight and at higher risk for chronic diseases like high blood pressure, heart disease, diabetes, and certain forms of cancer.

It seems like our whole lifestyle is engineered to sabotage our health, to make us fat and sick. According to a 2005 study, more than 40 percent of the TV ads aimed at kids were for candy, fast food, and snacks, and almost none for fresh fruit, vegetables, or seafood.

The restaurant industry pays lip service to good nutrition, but then often refuses to disclose nutritional information, and spends gazillions of dollars promoting heart-unhealthy saturated-fat-soaked food.

Personally, I think hamburgers are great. I like them so much I own several Fatburger restaurants myself, specializing in lean, juicy, old-fashioned burgers and trimmings. But meat is by no means the only ingredient in a healthy diet.

Food companies are dumping wildly excessive amounts of sodium into our prepared foods, fast food, and restaurant dishes—and a diet of too much sodium over time is linked to high blood pressure, which raises the risks of heart problems, stroke, and kidney disease.

Have you been to a Romano's Macaroni Grill restaurant lately? You might have ordered the Grilled Salmon Teriyaki, which sounds tasty and healthful. Care to know how much sodium is in your fish dish, including side orders? A mind-boggling 6,590 milligrams. That's almost three times the U.S. Dietary Guidelines recommended adult intake of sodium, 2,300 milligrams—*for an entire day*! For adults over fifty, African-Americans, and people who already suffer from high blood pressure, the recommended daily intake is 1,500 milligrams or less.

Even worse, a kid's Grilled Chicken & Broccoli at Romano's has 4,020 *milligrams of sodium!* That's for *kids!* Can you imagine the damage a steady diet of this kind of food would do to a child over the long term?

At least these guys put nutritional information on their Web site; you'll have no such luck if you go out to Applebee's, the self-described "largest casual dining concept in the world." If you want to find out how much saturated fat, trans fat, sugar, sodium, fiber, or calories are in any Applebee's item (except their Weight Watchers items), forget it. They won't tell you.

What's Applebee's excuse? Their Web site says, "With approximately 1,900 locations in the U.S. alone there are many different vendors, which makes it extremely difficult to obtain nutritional information for our items." My advice to them: figure it out. This is important stuff.

With this kind of lifestyle, it's no wonder we're packing on tons of weight and getting so sick.

It can sneak up on you, too. Listen to the story of a friend of mine, a marvelous lady and talented comedian named Poppi Kramer, who gradually gained a hundred pounds over the course of ten years.

When I was younger, I wasn't really considered fat, but I was on the pudgy-to-round side. And I felt the need to constantly lose weight. It was a constant yo-yo dieting way of life for me. When I went to college, I had a lot more time on my hands, which meant a lot more food on my plate, and I became about sixty pounds overweight.

When my dad was diagnosed with leukemia, I, like many other people, became an emotional eater. I ate until I probably put on another twenty pounds. I would get all sorts of take-out food, pizza, pasta, French fries. If I had a bag of something, I would eat the entire bag.

It kind of was like an avalanche. You start eating and eating and the more you eat, the less active you feel.

When my dad became healthy, I knew that I had to make a change. At five feet two, weighing 232 pounds is dangerous. I had hit my own personal rock bottom. . . .

I remember one day lying in my bed, and thinking, *Is the bed sinking?* And it was literally my fat, almost encompassing my neck like a tsunami!

But here's the great news: *you can turn it all around.* Poppi Kramer is living proof. She lost one hundred pounds of excess weight in one year, and won the national at-home *Biggest Loser* TV reality-show contest. Today, she looks and feels fantastic.

How did Poppi do it?

The *Biggest Loser* at Home contest gave me the tools to lose weight in the comfort of my own home. I was taught to work out every day. In addition to that, I had to watch my caloric intake.

I weighed and measured all my food and I kept a food journal. And I was religious about all of that.

When I started working out, I had to start by walking, but as I got stronger and in better shape, I was able to jog and then, gradually, run. Running became kind of a euphoric thing for me. It's the closest thing that I could feel to flying.

When I look back at the pants that I was wearing, almost one year ago today, it almost makes me cry. . . .

I always tell people, now I'm kind of like "Pure Poppi"; it's actually the version of me that I always knew was inside, but now it's on the outside. Before I did the show my mother looked at me and she said, "I just want the outside to match the inside," and that's what happened.

Notice one word Poppi didn't use? The D word. Diet.

DIETS NOT ONLY DON'T WORK—
DIETS MAKE YOU FAT

There's a new diet coming at us every single day. We're desperate to lose weight, but food is everywhere. Why cook when you can go out? Why walk when you can drive through? We're truly a fast-food nation.

Everybody you know seems to either be on a diet or is sick of having tried countless failed diets.

The very word "diet" bugs me. It bugs me because diets don't work.

In fact, diets make you fat.

During sixteen years of doing my TV show, I've discussed probably a thousand different types of diets—carrot diets, cabbage soup diets, lemonade diets, low-carb diets, high-protein diets.

Almost none of them works.

A diet is an easy quick fix. A diet is something that's written in a sound bite or condensed in a few pages to sound simple but really makes your whole life so much harder. It's something that makes you believe, "I have to have an answer today, a solution right now." The trouble is, that isn't how it works.

Have you heard of the Pickle Plus Diet weight-loss system? The key ingredients are pickles and salsa, which "speed up your metabolism" so you'll lose twenty pounds a month. For $15.95, you get a jar of pickles and a recipe book.

If you think this sounds far-fetched, you're right. It's a phony fad diet I made up as an experiment on my show. We set up hidden cameras and a sales booth at the Tri-County Flea Market on Long Island, hired an actress to pose as a sales rep, and started pitching the diet.

We wanted to see if people would actually fall for this hooey. Man, we hit the jackpot!

"Attention, shoppers" came the announcement on the speakers. "The new pickle diet has a booth set up on the second-floor jewelry exchange. Stop by to get free samples of their low-calorie pickles and their new salsa products!" In no time, our sales booth was swamped with customers checking out the Pickle Plus Diet.

Our customers were buzzing: "Yes, I want to go on the pickle diet!" "I saw the pickles, and I saw something that was gonna be helpful for my weight." "I love pickles. Any kind, any shape." "Yeah, it's gonna work because there's vinegar in there, and all this stuff that breaks down the fat." "I do love pickles. It's one of my weaknesses. You mean I could lose, like, one hundred pounds quick?"

Hundreds of people were jostling around our booth ready to plunk down $15.95, hoping to lose weight on a ridiculous phony diet!

Just now I typed the word "diet" into Google.

Care to guess how many hits I got? One hundred forty-seven million. That's 147,000,000. Don't you think if any of these diets actually worked they might have stopped at, oh, let's say 146,999,999?

Diets usually only focus on one piece of the puzzle—"don't eat potatoes" or "eat more protein," which is ridiculous. They're not focusing on the big picture, which has hundreds or thousands of pieces.

When you go on a diet, you think, *I have to eat less food. I've gotta give up my favorite foods. Certain things I can never eat again.* You do it because you're desperate. After two weeks or a month, you feel so deprived that you go back to your old way of eating and then you feel guilty.

Diets don't work because by definition they end. You cannot restrict yourself forever; it's too stressful, too hard. That's why diets are rarely seen to work beyond six months or a year.

In April 2007, the "Diets Don't Work" theory got a boost from researchers at the University of California at Los Angeles, who published a rigorous and comprehensive analysis of long-term diet studies in *American Psychologist*, the journal of the American Psychological Association.

"What happens to people on diets in the long run?" asked Traci Mann, UCLA associate professor of psychology and the lead author of the study. "We decided to dig up and analyze every study that followed people on diets for two to five years. We concluded most of them would have been better off not going on the diet at all."

At first, you can lose 5 to 10 percent of your weight on many diets, "but then the weight comes right back," said Mann. "We found that the majority of people regained all the weight, plus more. Sustained weight loss was found only in a small minority of participants, while complete weight regain was found in the majority. Diets do not lead to sustained weight loss or health benefits for the majority of people."

Even worse, the researchers found evidence that yo-yo dieting is linked to cardiovascular disease, stroke, diabetes, and altered immune system function. Their bottom line: "The benefits of dieting are too small and the potential harm is too large for dieting to be recommended as a safe, effective treatment for obesity."

Some people do lose weight for a while on one diet or another, and that's great for them. But the next time you hear your cousin-in-law rave about the twenty pounds he lost on the Maple Syrup and Hot Chili Pepper Diet or the Sugar Fast, or the next time a health-food store salesman tells you about a "clinically proven effective weight-loss pill," remember one stunning fact: not a single branded diet program or diet product has ever been proven in a large real-world scientific study among real people to significantly reduce weight and keep it off over the long term—three, or five, or ten years. It has never happened; 99.9 percent of the weight-loss marketing hype you see is pure, unadulterated bull.

Here's the big problem—scientists don't really know yet exactly how to get people to lose weight and make it stay off, outside of surgery. They're only in the very early stages of figuring this all out.

The truth is that the gold standard of diet research is the randomized controlled trial, but that's nearly impossible to do with food.

You can't get large groups of people to stick to a strict diet pattern over many years, much less to old age, so disease outcomes can be measured. As a result, there are hardly any such studies to rely on in planning our diets. Also, the research we do have on diets is muddy and imperfect. Much of it is based on studies that compare different populations, where you can't really disentangle actual causes and effects.

Scientists often study only one nutrient at a time. But the human diet is an almost infinitely complicated puzzle, and in the course of a day you eat hundreds or thousands of different nutrients and compounds in your food, in different combinations. The best experts on diet and nutrition will tell you that the truth is kind of a moving target and there's very little they know for sure.

On top of this, health experts change their minds as they get new information. Not long ago, many of them thought antioxidant supplements in pill form, such as vitamin E and beta-carotene, offered big health benefits. Now they say the research for this is weak to nonexistent, and since some antioxidant supplements may even have health risks, it's best to get these nutrients from whole foods instead. Experts used to stress low-fat diets. Now it turns out, some fats are good (omega-3s, polyunsaturated and monounsaturated fats), and some are bad (trans fats and saturated fats).

So what's the answer?

How are we supposed to figure this out?

In a world of unhealthy food choices, diets that don't work, and confusing nutritional information, how can we possibly make the right choices to live and eat well?

Well, I've got some fantastic news for you. . . .

The Living Well Code

How would you like to feel fantastic, lose weight, live longer and healthier, and cut your risk of many life-threatening diseases, including cardiovascular disease, the biggest killer of all?

I have discovered a formula that will help you and me achieve this dream.

It is not a pill, or a secret ingredient, or a ridiculous program based on cutting out entire food groups or impossible food schedules or starving yourself.

It is a subtle makeover of the life you are already living, a beautiful pattern of adjustments and new behaviors that are within your reach right now.

It is a new way of enjoying every second of your life.

This is huge news. It is history-changing and it is life-changing.

This has the power to revolutionize your health—and help you be physically reborn.

This literally has the power to save your life and the lives of your loved ones.

This formula is based on something magnificent that is starting to happen in the world of health and nutrition: the best experts around the world are piecing together thousands of different theories, laboratory experiments, and research studies, and they are starting to agree on many of the key points of what it takes to fight major diseases, achieve a healthy body weight, and truly Live Well.

By the way, when I say "experts," I'm not talking about self-described health gurus, or doctors or nutritionists with shaky credentials who happen to have a diet book on the market hyping a secret ingredient or a restrictive diet program.

I'm not talking about experts you'll find only in health-food stores or on the Internet. I'm talking about leading scientists, medical doctors, dietitians, and university researchers who publish their findings in peer-reviewed medical journals. These are people who study health and nutrition for a living, who base their ideas on real science.

I will introduce you to some of them soon, so you'll hear their ideas in their own words, talking to you directly.

These experts are coming together to support a series of simple, clear, real-world guidelines that have a huge potential payoff for your health and well-being.

I call it the Living Well Code.

The Living Well Code is not a punishing set of rules but a pattern of behaviors to aspire to and enjoy.

It is based on a new breakthrough insight in the scientific and medical communities: *the exact same steps that will help you achieve a healthy weight will also help you fight the risks of many major chronic diseases.*

The Living Well Code is a complete biological action package. It changed my life, and it can change yours, too.

THE LIVING WELL CODE

7 Simple Steps
to Supercharge Your Health
and Be Physically Reborn

1. Base your diet on a foundation of a rich variety of many different vegetables and fruits—especially in their fresh, natural, and whole states.

2. Include healthy carbohydrates from whole grains, and healthy fats and protein from foods like fish, beans, and nuts.

3. Minimize saturated and trans fats, sodium, processed foods, added sugars, and cholesterol in your diet.

4. Be mindful of your calories in and calories out, to work toward a healthy body weight.

5. Don't skip meals, deprive yourself, or go on fad diets.

6. Get regular physical activity, at least thirty to sixty minutes of moderate exercise on most days of the week.

7. Combine these steps and you can reduce your risk of many major diseases, such as:
   • cardiovascular disease
   • obesity
   • several forms of cancer
   • diabetes (type 2)
   • other diseases, including Alzheimer's disease, osteoarthritis, and macular degeneration

Note: If you eat meat and poultry, make them lean, and trim off visible fat. If you enjoy dairy products, make them nonfat or low-fat.

The Living Well Code is for you if you simply want to feel great in your daily life.

It is for you if you want to live a longer and healthier life, and reduce the risks of killer diseases like heart disease, obesity, and several forms of cancer.

And if you're fighting existing diseases like Parkinson's or multiple sclerosis, you can benefit by putting the Living Well Code into action in consultation with your doctor, because it can help keep your body in optimal overall health.

The Living Well Code is not fixed in stone for all time. It has a strong foundation in evidence, but it also is a living, organic thing that evolves and improves with new scientific debates and discoveries. The language above is my personal synthesis of the world's best expert opinions on Living Well as of today.

When you boil it all down, it's an extraordinarily simple formula. Notice I said "simple," not necessarily "easy," because I know how hard it can be to Live Well in a society that is so often geared to making us live poorly.

But in a world of bad diets, bogus health experts, and an infinity of conflicting and complex health information, the truth is really not that complicated at all. As Michael Pollan, the author of the excellent book *The Omnivore's Dilemma*, put it:

> **Eat food. Not too much. Mostly plants.**
> **That, more or less, is the short answer to the supposedly incredibly complicated and confusing question of what we humans should eat in order to be maximally healthy.**

You don't need to cleanse or detox or fast or starve yourself to start getting slim and healthy. You just need to start living the basic principles of the Code.

Sometimes, experts disagree on some of the exact wording of their versions of the Code.

Some insist on putting eggs on the list of good sources of healthy protein, while others object because they're high in cholesterol. Some experts love potatoes, while a few experts criticize them because of their "high glycemic index," which supposedly might contribute to weight gain. The list of diseases influenced by diet and exercise can change as new research comes in.

But the general foundations of what I call the Living Well Code are supported by experts affiliated with top universities and hospitals around the world and such institutions as the World Health Organization, the U.S. Department of Health and Human Services, the American Cancer Society, the American Heart Association, the American Diabetes

Association, the Alzheimer's Association, and the American Dietetic Association, to name just a few.

The Living Well Code should be your life mantra. You should read it out loud to yourself, your family, and your doctor. Stick a copy of it on your refrigerator, in your briefcase or purse, in your kid's lunchbox. Make it a screensaver on your computer.

It is your road map to fantastic health.

We've long heard that vegetables, fruits, and exercise are good for you. We've heard it so often from our moms, grandmoms, and health authorities that we're kind of numb to it.

"Hey, Montel, all right already—fruits and vegetables are good for you! We get it!"

But what's new is that only in the last few years have the experts realized the full impact of a stunning reality: *the right dietary pattern combined with exercise is a potent, powerful disease fighter.* In fact, the Living Well Code is so powerful that it should strike terror in the souls of our most bloodthirsty killers—heart disease, high blood pressure, obesity, and cancer.

It's important to point out that diet and exercise are not the answer to all illnesses. Millions of Americans get sick through absolutely no fault of their own, through genetic-only causes.

For example, the American Cancer Society estimates that only one-third of cancers are related to diet and activity factors. But the flip side of that is that Living Well—eating healthy, having a healthy body weight, and getting regular physical activity—may help lower your risks for a number of killer forms of cancer, including cancers of the lung, stomach, breast, gallbladder, thyroid, ovaries, and colon, among others.

Diets don't work—but healthy eating does.

The everyday food you put in your body can literally kill you.

But the healthy food you put in your body, and the exercise you do, can fight disease and transform your body into a masterpiece of power and energy.

Sound too good to be true? Well, it *is* good, and it is absolutely true.

A LIFE-CHANGING SERIES
OF INSIGHTS ON HOW YOU CAN LIVE WELL

In 2005, two scientists at the University of California–Los Angeles (UCLA) physiology department, Christian K. Roberts, Ph.D., and R. James Barnard, Ph.D., published an extraordinary article called "Effects of Exercise and Diet on Chronic Disease" in a scientific journal called the *Journal of Applied Physiology*. It's a seventeen-page article with 424 footnotes. You can look it up for yourself on the Internet.

The article isn't exactly light beach reading. It's fairly dense and technical. It's basically an attempt to capture and summarize all the best scientific evidence on the connections between diet, exercise, and chronic disease. But it could be the most important article you'll ever read. It should be required reading for every person, every doctor, and every health expert and alleged health guru in the world. It's like an owner's manual for your body and how you can transform your physical destiny.

Good science is like a Sherlock Holmes mystery: it takes tough, smart detective work. For their analysis, Professors Roberts and Barnard reviewed hundreds of the best studies on diet, exercise, and health from around the world, sifted the good evidence from the bad, and searched for key insights, trends, patterns, and clues in a blizzard of data.

They found these insights in a series of landmark health and medical studies conducted over the decades, including the Seven Countries Study, the Framingham Heart Study, the Lyon Diet Heart Study, the Nurses' Health Study, the Health Professionals Follow-up Study, the Dietary Approaches to Stop Hypertension (DASH) Trial, the EPIC study (European Prospective Investigation into Cancer and Nutrition), and the Diabetes Prevention Program.

In their report, Roberts and Barnard revealed the scope of the problem in stark terms:

• Most chronic diseases today can be linked to inappropriate diets and physical inactivity.

- The leading killers in Westernized society are cardiovascular diseases (like coronary artery disease, hypertension, stroke, and heart failure), type 2 diabetes, metabolic syndrome (a combination of symptoms that increase the risk of cardiovascular diseases), and cancer.
- Overweight and obesity (a BMI, or body mass index greater than 25) are present in 60 percent of the adult U.S. population and obesity and diabetes are now common in children.
- Inactivity and diet will soon rank as the number-one cause of death in the United States.
- Since more than 55 percent of American adults don't engage in regular physical activity, and more than 75 percent do not eat at least five fruits and vegetables a day, "it is no surprise that chronic diseases are the most common cause of preventable death in the United States."

The solutions identified by Professors Roberts and Barnard are, in my opinion, astonishing. And when you boil them all down, they are elegantly simple.

This is what they found:

- Evidence that "the vast majority of chronic disease may be prevented" when daily physical activity of one hour is performed in combination with "a natural food diet, high in fiber-containing fruits, vegetables, and whole grains, and naturally low in fat, containing abundant amounts of vitamins, minerals, and phytochemicals." The evidence supporting this approach for both the prevention and the treatment of major diseases, they wrote, is "overwhelming."
- Specifically, "the evidence is overwhelming that physical activity and diet can reduce the risk of developing numerous chronic diseases, including CAD [coronary artery disease], hypertension, diabetes, metabolic syndrome, and several forms of cancer, and in many cases in fact reverse existing disease."

- Additionally, they concluded, the risk of other major chronic diseases may be lowered by physical activity and diet, including osteoarthritis, osteoporosis, stroke and congestive heart failure, chronic renal failure, Alzheimer's disease, and, *ahem*, erectile dysfunction.

These three bullets are close to a holy grail of Living Well.

Notice the bold language the scientists used, words like "the vast majority of chronic disease may be prevented," "the evidence is overwhelming," "reverse existing disease." That's extremely powerful stuff.

These are some of the most exciting medical ideas I've ever seen—because you don't need an operation or a prescription to put them into action and start reaping the benefits; all you need is a grocery store or farmers' market and a pair of sneakers!

You may think your genes are the main trigger of illness, but, in fact, Professors Roberts and Barnard point out, many chronic diseases are largely the result of interactions between your genes and your environment. Genes can predispose you to illness, but environmental factors like diet and lifestyle can often trigger diseases to manifest themselves.

A big lesson from our genes is that you and I inherited a genome that is literally programmed for daily physical activity and a high-fiber diet.

In other words, you and I are genetically programmed to follow the Living Well Code.

Here are three big reasons for us to follow the Living Well Code:

- **The Living Well Code unleashes the power of the ultimate super-foods.**
- **The Living Well Code can help you lose weight and keep it off.**
- **The Living Well Code can help you live longer and feel better by fighting a wide array of major diseases.**

LET'S TALK ABOUT SEX

Can the Living Well Code heat up your sex life?

The research is preliminary, but it just might.

In the U.S., erectile dysfunction (ED) affects up to 30 million men, and up to 52 percent of men between the ages of forty and seventy. Additionally, millions of American women suffer from some form of sexual dysfunction.

It turns out that some of the hottest new research on the possible connections among diet, physical activity, and sex is coming out of one of the world's sexiest countries: Italy. The research is being performed by Dr. Katherine Esposito of the University of Naples and her colleagues; it is based on both population studies and small interventional trial studies with men and women. Here are some of their key recent observations and findings:

- Obesity may be a risk factor for sexual dysfunction in both sexes. Sexual problems in both men and women are influenced by both health-related and psychosocial factors.
- Physical activity and leanness are associated with a reduced risk for ED.
- Obesity, hypertension, smoking, and diabetes are significantly associated with ED risk. Improvement of these risk factors may ameliorate the burden of ED.
- Dietary factors may be important in developing ED: adoption of healthy eating patterns would hopefully help prevent ED.
- One-third of obese men with ED can regain their sexual activity after adopting healthy lifestyle behaviors, mainly regular exercise and reducing weight.
- Adopting a healthy lifestyle is strongly recommended in order to reduce the prevalence of the metabolic syndrome and hence the burden of ED.
- A Mediterranean-style diet rich in whole grains, fruits, vegetables, nuts, and olive oil might be effective in improving sexual function in both men and women with metabolic syndrome.

It looks like Living Well may be a powerful tool for a richer, more pleasurable and fulfilling sex life, for both you and your partner.

How's that for an awesome benefit?

COME WITH ME ON A LIVING WELL FIELD TRIP

Let's go on a fantastic journey together, you and I.

Let's go to the supermarket.

Bring along your kids or your partner if you like.

A lot of people race past the produce section on their way to the packaged food, frozen dinners, chips, and soda.

Huge mistake!

The fruit and vegetable aisles are the richest section of the store. You should be spending lots of your quality shopping time here.

Today, let's stop and slowly look around and admire the piles of fruits and veggies.

Immerse yourself in the fruits and veggies. They are your physical salvation.

Let your eyes drink in the dazzling shades, the Picasso shapes and van Gogh colors. Admire the electric oranges and yellows of the citrus fruits, the Day-Glo green shades of the leafy greens, the rich purple of the eggplants, and the intoxicating bursts of aroma from the fresh herbs.

Now close your eyes and think of some words of wisdom from the Bible, words that Genesis 1:29 attributes to God:

> **Behold, I have given you every herb bearing seed, which is upon the face of all the earth, and every tree, in the which is the fruit of a tree yielding seed; to you it shall be for meat.**

To me, this means God is telling us to load up on veggies, fruits, and herbs, and to enjoy a plant-based, whole-foods diet. They are loving gifts from God, and nature, and Mother Earth. Take a deep breath and feel your heart beating. It's beating largely because of those plants in the produce pile—they are your life force.

I love going to the grocery store. Sometimes I'll go to the vegetable bins and just stand there and look around. There are few places in the world where you can see this much of nature's variety in one place. I'll go down the aisles with my cart and grab a bundle and a bundle and a bundle. They are a symphony of nature, and they're all little master-pieces of designs, flavors, and ingredients.

Grab a fresh, ripe, juicy peach and hold it up to the light. Check this ravishing beauty out. Never in a million years could Albert Einstein him-self figure out how to create something this glorious.

I'm a "flexitarian"—that is, I eat an intensely plant-based diet, but I also enjoy fish, eggs, and steak. I am also a man who as a special treat loves a good juicy cheeseburger made from top-quality lean beef. But on a day-to-day basis, the real superstar of my diet is the stuff you'll find in the produce section.

Vegetables and fruits are the ultimate superfoods.

In a world of alleged superfoods, vegetables and fruits are truly in a class by themselves. Vegetables and fruits, along with whole grains, are among the hottest superstars in the world of nutrition.

Vegetables and fruits are the new "smart drugs," offering a wide range of potential benefits and no known side effects. In 2005, the U.S. Departments of Health and Human Services and Agriculture published the "Dietary Guidelines for Americans," an expert report that summa-rized their health benefits:

- **Disease-fighting benefit:** "Greater consumption of fruits and vegetables (5 to 13 servings or 2½ to 6½ cups per day depending on calorie needs) is associated with a reduced risk of stroke and perhaps other cardiovas-cular diseases, with a reduced risk of cancers in certain sites (oral cavity and pharynx, larynx, lung, esophagus, stomach, and colon-rectum), and with a reduced risk of type 2 diabetes (vegetables more than fruit)."

- **Weight-loss benefit:** "Increased consumption of fruits and vegetables may be a useful component of programs designed to achieve and sustain weight loss."

How does a diet rich in vegetables and fruits fight disease and help you lose weight?

There are two short answers:

- **High Nutrient Density:** Fruits and vegetables contain health-promoting phytochemicals, antioxidants, fiber, vitamins, minerals, and nutrients, which all combine to fight disease and promote health.
- **Low Calorie Density:** Fruits and vegetables have low "calories-per-bite" and high fiber and water content, which promote fullness and healthy weight, while displacing less healthy, higher-calorie foods.

But specifically, how does all this work and what is the precise sequence of action? There are many theories, but the experts aren't really sure.

The evidence strongly suggests that a vegetable-and-fruit-rich diet promotes health, but no one is exactly sure why. A piece of fruit may look simple, but it is actually a magnificently complicated chemical package that scientists are only starting to figure out.

One recent theory is that rather than containing one, or two, or five magic bullets, there may in fact be many hundreds or thousands of exquisitely complex chemical interactions in vegetables and fruits that work together in a vast symphony to promote health.

It will take many years, or even decades, before scientists fully unlock the mystery. For now, we have speculation and educated opinions.

"Disease prevention might not be attributable to single nutrients, but to the interaction of nutrient and non-nutritive components in whole foods," wrote Dr. Lyn Steffen of the University of Minnesota School of Public Health, in the medical journal the *Lancet* in 2004. "It is likely that the combination of nutrients and compounds in foods has greater health benefits than the individual nutrient alone."

"The easiest advice," said Dr. Ritva Butrum, senior science adviser to the American Institute for Cancer Research, "is to cut down on animal products and eat a diet that is mostly made up of many brightly colored vegetables and fruits, along with whole grains and beans." There are so many health-protective substances in these foods, said Dr. Butrum, that scientists estimate eating a large variety every day can lower the risk of cancer by at least 20 percent.

Here is a rundown on many of the benefits you can enjoy from veggies and fruits, according to the most recent U.S. Dietary Guidelines:

- Eating a diet rich in fruits and vegetables as part of an overall healthy diet may reduce risk for stroke and perhaps other cardiovascular diseases.
- Eating a diet rich in fruits and vegetables as part of an overall healthy diet may reduce risk for type 2 diabetes.
- Eating a diet rich in fruits and vegetables as part of an overall healthy diet may protect against certain cancers, such as mouth, stomach, and colon-rectum cancer.
- Diets rich in foods containing fiber, such as fruits and vegetables, may reduce the risk of coronary heart disease.
- Eating fruits and vegetables rich in potassium as part of an overall healthy diet may reduce the risk of developing kidney stones and may help to decrease bone loss.
- Eating foods such as vegetables that are low in calories per cup instead of some other higher-calorie food may be useful in helping to lower calorie intake.
- Most vegetables are naturally low in fat and calories. None have cholesterol. (Sauces or seasonings may add fat, calories, or cholesterol.)
- Vegetables are important sources of many nutrients, including

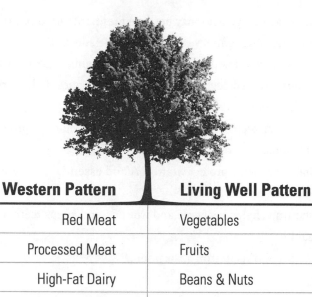

Western Pattern	Living Well Pattern
Red Meat	Vegetables
Processed Meat	Fruits
High-Fat Dairy	Beans & Nuts
Butter	Fish/Seafood
Refined Grains	Whole Grains
Processed & Packaged Foods	Whole & Natural Foods

potassium, dietary fiber, folate (folic acid), vitamin A, vitamin E, and vitamin C.

- Diets rich in potassium may help to maintain healthy blood pressure. Vegetable sources of potassium include sweet potatoes, white potatoes, white beans, tomato products (paste, sauce, and juice), beet greens, soybeans, lima beans, winter squash, spinach, lentils, kidney beans, and split peas.

- Dietary fiber from vegetables, as part of an overall healthy diet, helps reduce blood cholesterol levels and may lower risk of heart disease. Fiber is important for proper bowel function. It helps reduce constipation and diverticulosis. Fiber-containing foods such as vegetables help provide a feeling of fullness with fewer calories.

- Folate (folic acid) helps the body form red blood cells. Women of childbearing age who may become pregnant and those in the first trimester of pregnancy should consume adequate folate, including folic acid from fortified foods or supplements. This reduces the risk of neural tube defects, spina bifida, and anencephaly during fetal development.

- Vitamin A keeps eyes and skin healthy and helps to protect against infections.
- Vitamin E helps protect vitamin A and essential fatty acids from cell oxidation.
- Vitamin C helps heal cuts and wounds and keeps teeth and gums healthy.
- Vitamin C aids in iron absorption.

How can we put all this knowledge to work in our own lives? How can we translate the Living Well Code into a living reality in our world of impossible schedules, stress, and frantic family life?

Just give me 21 days . . . and you and I can change your life.

PART II: THE 21-DAY LIVING WELL PROGRAM

Introduction

I **want you to transform your life.**

I want you to supercharge your health.

I want you to live longer and healthier.

I want your doctor to smile in amazement at how well you're doing at your checkups.

And I want you to feel spectacular.

Hey, these are really ambitious goals!

But that's the only kind of goal I believe in.

It is a beautiful dream, and together, you and I can make it a flesh-and-blood reality.

This 21-Day Living Well Program is designed to power up your nutrition and get you moving more—two critical steps that will give you a strong start on the path to these goals, if you stick with them for the long term.

You and I are living in an incredibly exciting time! Many of the most distinguished doctors and scientists around the world are coming together in support of the foundations of the Living Well Code, which may help you reduce your risks for diseases like cardiovascular disease, obesity, several forms of cancer, diabetes (type 2), Alzheimer's disease, osteoarthritis, and macular degeneration.

Think about it—that's an amazing package of benefits!

This program is about putting the Living Well Code into action.

Why did I choose 21 days to start you on this path?

Because 21 days is how long it can take to change a habit. And one of the keys to Living Well is to take small, achievable steps, and faithfully track your progress.

You set a 21-day goal about losing some weight and getting yourself in shape. And once you accomplish one goal, then you're going to accomplish the next and the next and the next. And you're on the road to success. A few small steps at a time.

I don't like quick fixes. They usually don't work. Take diets, for example. There are tons of diets out there that promise things like "rapid weight loss," or "21 Pounds in 21 Days." But that doesn't translate to long-term health, and chances are that these kinds of diets will backfire.

Any diet can help you lose weight, and even quickly, if it cuts your daily calorie intake. But you'll probably fall off the diet at some point and wind up putting on more weight. Diets make you fat—it's true!

Let's take small steps together, you and I.

Let's take good solid baby steps, not dangerous leaps.

I want you to feel for yourself that with every little change you make and every goal you achieve, it gets to be almost habit-forming.

Let's get started over the course of 21 days, and let's look at the end of our twenty-first day as a beginning, not an end.

Here's how it works: three weeks, two small steps per week:

Week 1: Add in the Green Power
Small Steps:
- Add more vegetables and fruits to your diet, especially in their fresh, natural, and whole forms.
- Add whole grains and fish to your diet.

Week 2: Energize Your Body
Small Steps:

- Be mindful of your calories in and calories out to work toward a healthy body weight.
- Gradually begin working toward the target of at least thirty to sixty minutes of moderate physical activity on most days of the week.

Week 3: Start to Live Well for Life
Small Steps:

- Start switching in healthier choices, and minimizing saturated and trans fats, sodium, processed foods, added sugars, and cholesterol from your diet.
- Start adopting healthy lifetime attitudes, like not skipping meals or going on fad diets, and building a protective home environment for your family.

Eating right and getting regular physical activity is a lifetime process. It's how to train for the sport of life.

Forget the fad diet books, forget the cheesy ads, and forget the sales hype. You're never going to make a change in anything important in your life unless it starts way down inside you, deep in your heart. Those are the types of changes that will last a lifetime.

No matter where you are in life, if you can make a few key changes, you can make a huge difference in your whole world.

You'll find that once you really commit yourself to change, the whole world works with you.

I want you to write your ideas and checkmarks on the pages that follow, and mark them up with circles and underlines.

Okay, come on—*Let's go!*

Add in the Green Power

Small Steps:

- Add more vegetables and fruits to your diet, especially in their fresh, natural, and whole forms.
- Add whole grains and fish to your diet.

Take a Self-Snapshot of Your Feelings and Goals

Take a deep, relaxing breath.

Feel yourself breathe, feel your heart beating, your blood pumping, and your brain cells crackling.

I want you to start thinking about what it is to be truly healthy. To live better.

This is our first day on the road to Living Well.

The next 21 days will be action-packed, challenging, and, I hope, fun.

Look, I'm not just rooting for you—I'm dancing, whooping, and hollering for you!

One of my greatest joys in life is when I discover how people have improved their lives based on something I've said, written, or presented on my show. You wouldn't believe how often I hear these stories as I walk through my life and meet people on the street and in airports, and let me tell you, there are few sweeter feelings in life.

Today, on Day 1, let's see where you are, and where you want to go.

Then let's start making some specific, achievable Action Plans to get there.

Before starting this or any other nutrition or exercise plan, you should see your doctor.

He or she should test your health stats, like blood pressure, weight, and cholesterol, advise you on special concerns and medications (especially if you're a woman of childbearing age, or pregnant, or have a health condition), refer you to specialists or dietitians if necessary, and customize a health plan for you. Show this book to your doctor and talk it over.

Next, at home, I want you to strip your clothes off.

You heard me—take 'em off!

Stand in front of a mirror in your underpants.

Take some pictures of your whole body—side views and frontal. Then file the pictures away and forget them for a while.

Now ask yourself how you feel physically, and rate yourself on this 1-to-10 scale by checking off a number:

HOW DO YOU FEEL PHYSICALLY RIGHT NOW?

	Check One
• **I feel a Magnificent 10:** I can conquer the world, run a marathon, and dance all night. I am invincible.	_____ 10
• **I feel a Good to Very Good 6–9:**	
I feel OK but want to feel my best.	_____ 9
	_____ 8
	_____ 7
	_____ 6
• **I feel a So-So 5:**	
I was in good shape until a few years ago, but now I'm overweight and I get winded easily.	_____ 5
• **I feel a Bad to Fair 2–4:**	
I really don't feel that good. I've got to feel much healthier.	_____ 4
	_____ 3
	_____ 2
• **I am a Really Lousy 1:**	
I'm exhausted all the time, I'm fat, and I'm sweaty. At this rate, I'll probably get sick, with something like chest pains, a heart attack, or diabetes. This is totally ridiculous.	_____ 1

By the way, before I started my own personal Living Well regimen, I averaged about a day-to-day 5 or 6. These days, after factoring in my MS symptoms, now that I'm truly Living Well, I usually feel at an 8, 9, or 10. Not bad at all.

LET'S DISCOVER YOUR LIVING WELL TARGET WEIGHT

Next let's measure a very important stat—your body mass index, or BMI. Your BMI is a widely used indicator of your body weight in relation to your height, a measurement that is connected to your risk of disease and death. This is an excellent starting point on the journey to Living Well—to work toward a healthy body weight.

According to the National Institutes of Health, extra weight can put you at higher risk for type 2 diabetes (high blood sugar), high blood pressure, high cholesterol, heart disease and stroke, some types of cancer, sleep apnea (when breathing stops for short periods during sleep), osteoarthritis (wearing away of the joints), gallbladder disease, irregular periods, and problems with pregnancy.

The great news is that a weight loss of 5 to 15 percent of body weight may improve your health and quality of life, and prevent these health problems. For a person who weighs two hundred pounds, that means losing ten to thirty pounds. Experts also agree that you may gain health benefits from even a *small* weight loss if:

- you are obese based on your BMI;
- you are overweight based on your BMI and have weight-related health problems or a family history of such problems; or
- you have a waist that measures more than forty inches if you are a man or more than thirty-five inches if you are a woman.

Here's a really important point: most experts consider a weight-loss rate of one or two pounds a week to be healthy and sustainable. *Any more than that is not recommended.*

A crash diet or fad diet may promise much faster weight loss, but there are health risks with too-rapid weight loss, plus the high probability that you'll quickly gain it all back and more. Next time you see a fad diet book promising "21 Pounds in 21 Days," skip it. One to two pounds a week is the healthy way to lose extra pounds.

Use the chart below to estimate your BMI. Find your weight on the bottom of the graph. Go straight up from that point until you come to the line that matches your height.

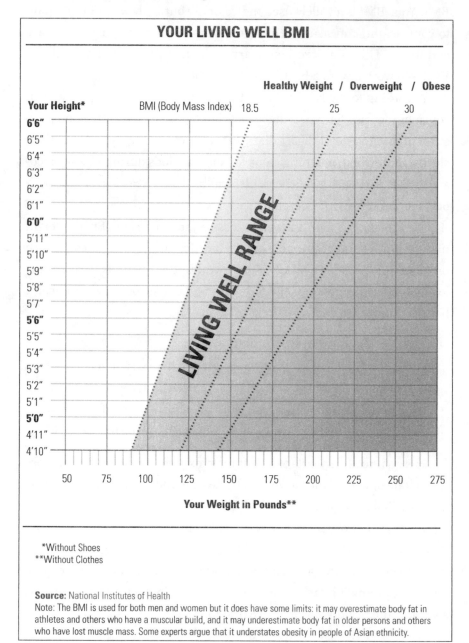

YOUR LIVING WELL BMI

Healthy Weight / Overweight / Obese

Your Height*   BMI (Body Mass Index)   18.5   25   30

*Without Shoes
**Without Clothes

Source: National Institutes of Health
Note: The BMI is used for both men and women but it does have some limits: it may overestimate body fat in athletes and others who have a muscular build, and it may underestimate body fat in older persons and others who have lost muscle mass. Some experts argue that it understates obesity in people of Asian ethnicity.

If your BMI is:	You are:
Below 18.5	Underweight
Between 18.5 and 24.9	At a Living Well Healthy Weight. Congratulations! This is the range where you want to be.
Between 25.0 and 29.9	Overweight
30.0 and Above	Obese

LET'S WRITE DOWN YOUR ACHIEVABLE LONG-TERM GOALS FOR LIVING WELL

Next, let's think about setting some long-term goals that are realistic and sustainable.

Run through this list, check off the goals you most strongly desire and think you could realistically achieve (be bold—be ambitious!), and fill in your additional goals at the bottom. Check off and write the goals in ink right on this page in the book so you can refer back to them in the weeks and months ahead.

- I want to walk up a flight of stairs without getting winded. _____
- I want to chase my kids around the yard for an hour without feeling exhausted. _____
- I want my partner to gawk at me and say, "Damn, you look good!" _____
- I want to be able to fast walk three miles and feel excellent. _____
- I want to shrink these stupid love handles I'm lugging around my belly. _____
- I want my skin to look better. _____
- I want to live longer than my parents. _____
- I want to feel powerful, strong, and packed with energy. _____
- I want to be more productive at work. _____
- I want to look smokin'-hot at my class reunion. _____

- I want to fit into the clothes that got too tight for me. _____
- I want the physical ability to enjoy more pleasurable sex. _____
- I want to enjoy food and get full, instead of stuffing myself into a semi-coma. _____
- I want to live longer by cutting my risks for chronic diseases like heart disease and diabetes. _____
- I want my doctor to give me good marks on blood pressure and cholesterol. _____
- I want to help my kids feel and look great and healthy. _____
- I just want a flatter belly. _____
- I just want to feel healthy. _____
- I'd like to lose one to two pounds per week over the course of a few months. _____
- I want to parade around the beach in a string bikini or Speedo. _____
- I want to go from overweight to a healthy, normal weight. _____
- I just want to look in the mirror and be happy with what I see. _____
- _____ _____
- _____ _____
- _____ _____
- _____ _____
- _____ _____

Incidentally, a Speedo isn't usually my style, but I'm telling you, I can get away with it at age fifty-one!

Finally, today and every day for the rest of this week, I want you to fill out this Living Well Action Plan. Our goals this week are to Add in the Green Power, which means bringing more of the earth's healthiest foods into our diet: veggies and fruits, whole grains and fish.

Every day, jot down all the food you eat, including snacks and liquid candy (sugared soft drinks). Jot down all the physical activity you do, everything from household chores and routine walking to structured exercise.

LIVING WELL ACTION PLAN

WEEK 1
ADD IN THE GREEN POWER

Small Steps:
- Start adding many different vegetables and fruits to your diet, especially in their fresh, natural and whole forms.

- Start adding whole grains and fish to your diet.

	MON	TUE	WED	THU	FRI	SAT	SUN
BREAKFAST							
LUNCH							
DINNER							
ALL OTHER: *Snacks, Lattes, Candy, Liquid Candy (Sugared Beverages), Office Munchies, etc.*							
PHYSICAL ACTIVITY TYPE:							
HOW MANY MINUTES:							

MY SPECIFIC PLANS TO LIVE WELL THIS WEEK:

The kinds of foods I'll enjoy:

The physical activities I'll enjoy:

The behaviors I'll make better:

The attitudes I'll make better:

Ways I'll help my family live well:

What if you could sit down with the greatest, most distinguished health experts and ask them what the secrets are to lose weight, fight disease, live longer, and feel fantastic?

That's exactly what I've done for you in this 21-day program.

I reached out to the "best of the best" nutrition, fitness, and diet experts around the country and asked them to tell us how to Live Well.

This is a super–summit meeting of the greatest brains on healthy living. They are a powerful, incredibly accomplished, insatiably curious, enthusiastic, and elite group of the most respected doctors and scientists in their fields.

I asked each one to step up and talk to us directly about their most important lessons, insights, theories, and research findings.

I think you'll be as amazed as I am that so much of what they have to say provides strong support for the foundations of the Living Well Code. You'll notice that their insights often overlap and build on each other.

I want you to read these expert comments thoroughly, because they offer such powerful insights to make us healthier and happier.

Their opinions are so important, I think you should read them aloud to your family over the breakfast or dinner table.

LIVING WELL EXPERT
Walter Willett M.D.

Dr. Walter Willett is the chairman of the department of nutrition at the Harvard School of Public Health and a professor of medicine at the Harvard Medical School.

I'm especially thrilled to hear Dr. Willett's opinions, because he is considered one of the "deans" of diet and nutrition research.

Dr. Willett, the author of the book *Eat, Drink, and Be Healthy: The Harvard Medical School Guide to Healthy Eating*, is a leader in the landmark Nurses' Health Study and Health Professionals Follow-up Study.

He is also a leader in the campaign to get harmful trans fats out of our nation's food supply.

I love what Dr. Willett has to say about food variety and healthy eating, and about how fantastic it makes you feel. That's been a big lesson in my own life.

The topic of nutrition and health is inherently complicated, even for someone working in the field on a day-to-day basis like I do.

Sometimes there are leaps in knowledge that are not confirmed. Science is often two steps forward, one step backward, and one step sideways.

But actually, there has been a lot of emerging consensus among people working in the area of nutrition and health that there are some key elements of a healthy diet. They are simple and straightforward, but put together they make a huge impact.

Tip #1: Get plenty of fruits and vegetables into your diet.

Tip #2: Switch from unhealthy fats (trans fat and saturated fat) to healthier fats (monounsaturated and polyunsaturated fats).

Tip #3: Get healthy forms of carbohydrate in your diet—replace refined starches and sugars with whole grains.

These three simple messages will have a huge positive impact on your health.

Then if you add healthy sources of protein, and get regular physical activity, you'll see a huge impact on not just heart disease, but diabetes and many other outcomes as well.

I don't think there is anybody who would disagree with these three core messages. Some people may describe them slightly differ-

(continued)

ently from others, but I think everybody will sign on to these three basic points as being fundamentally important.

Some of this is happening already without people being aware of it. The healthier types of fat are coming into our diet. The labeling of trans fat is now required, and manufacturers and restaurants are getting trans fat out of their foods. So, almost invisibly there's been a change for the better in our food supply.

Whole grains are coming into our diet more slowly, but compared to ten years ago, there are many more whole grain products available in any grocery store.

We've made slower progress in getting people to eat more fruits and vegetables. It's the toughest, because it is not just a cultural change but involves real issues of cost and availability for many people.

Unfortunately the cheapest ingredients for the food industry are refined starch and sugar and partially hydrogenated vegetable oil. There are all kinds of products, particularly in fast food, that are crafted out of those three basic ingredients, creating some of the unhealthiest calories you can eat, and the biggest profits for the food industry.

But you can eat very well on a limited budget. A lot of people think you have to spend a lot of money to eat well. It's really not true.

We showed in *Eat, Drink, and Be Healthy* that one person can eat very enjoyably for just $2.64 per day. You just have to plan and think a little bit more about what you're doing.

We reviewed some of the research on raw foods, and we couldn't see that it really made much difference whether food is raw or not. In many instances, frozen food and sometimes even in a few instances canned food can actually be better. Produce has often been picked, shipped, and stored over the course of weeks before it gets to our supermarkets, possibly losing nutrients along the way. Something that's flash-frozen within a couple hours of picking is going to be better preserved.

Virtually no one can stay with an extreme diet for a long time. In many cases an extreme diet will be unhealthy and unbalanced. The real issue is to find a way to eat well for a lifetime, to eat a variety of flavors and tastes, so that it is something that you can stay with for a lifetime.

Eating well not only has a huge impact on your overall health, and on your cancer or heart disease twenty years from now—it has a huge impact on how you feel and enjoy life every day.

What surprised me the most about writing *Eat, Drink, and Be Healthy* was the e-mails and letters I got from readers saying, "Thank you. This has changed my life." "I feel so much better now." "I feel like I'm in control, my blood sugar is down, my cholesterol is down," and "I just have more energy and feel good about myself."

That's incredibly important to understand.

If you've never eaten healthy and exercised regularly, you'll feel so much better when you do. ■

Eat the Rainbow: The Top 10 Living Well Powerhouse Foods

I **f you're used to buying lots of processed foods, soda, and snacks for your family, today I want you to start thinking about gradually shifting instead toward buying more natural whole foods—foods that are closer to the way the earth made them.**

I want you to think of the supermarket in a slightly new way.

I want you to think of the produce section as the main attraction of your shopping trip, and think about the aisles full of frozen dinners, cookies, ice cream, liquid candy (sugar-sweetened soda), crackers, and other processed foods as very occasional or unnecessary destinations.

What should we buy at the supermarket?

We hear about superfoods all the time—one week it's goji berries, the next it's pomegranate juice, and then it's acai berries.

But, in fact, the idea of a few superfoods is misleading.

A healthy diet is not based on a few supposed superfoods, but instead on long-term healthy eating patterns, starring lots of fruits and vegetables, whole grains, fish, and other healthy sources of good fats, good carbohydrates, and protein.

Within that context, however, there are some fantastic foods and food categories that stand out as elite choices, because they are extra-rich in nutrients per bite. I call them the Top 10 Living Well Powerhouse Foods:

1. Rainbow Foods—all Veggies and Fruits
2. Antioxidant Superstars
3. Superpower Greens: Leafy and Cruciferous Veggies
4. Whole Grains
5. SuperFish
6. Extra-Virgin Olive Oil
7. Canola Oil
8. Nuts
9. Sweet Potatoes
10. Custom-Bottled Personal Ice Water

The categories can overlap, and this is not a list of all nutritious foods by any means, but you should start welcoming fantastic foods like these into your diet as a key foundation of Living Well.

Note: When you're adding more veggies and fruits to your diet, it's a good idea to do it gradually over the course of a few weeks, to give your body time to adjust.

1. RAINBOW FOODS: Think of your diet as a painting you create every day, and splash it with a dazzling array of bold, rich colors from a variety of fruits and vegetables. Next time you're at a salad bar, the supermarket, or a farmers' market, pretend you're Jackson Pollock and splash on the superhealthy colors.

Phytochemicals are natural compounds found in fruits, veggies, and plants that help give them colors, and they also may help us fight disease, especially when they are working in combination. Thousands of phytochemicals have been discovered so far, and one group called flavonoids has an estimated five thousand phytochemicals alone. Scientists are just now beginning to figure out the health-promoting properties of phyto-chemicals.

"Each individual phytochemical has its own function in protecting us against disease," said Melanie Polk, the director of nutrition educa-tion at the American Institute for Cancer Research (AICR). "One way of getting a good variety of these protective phytochemicals is to eat a whole rainbow of colors."

I'm including beans in the Rainbow Foods veggie category, because they're good, cheap, meatless sources of protein, fiber, potassium, folate, and iron. The government's Dietary Guidelines for Americans urge us to eat at least three cups of legumes (beans, peas, and lentils) a week.

When buying canned veggies and fruit, look for little or no sodium or added sugar.

Think of the whole category of fruits and vegetables as the ultimate superfoods.

Don't worry about what the latest trendy antioxidant or "food of the moment" is. Fruits and veggies are great low-fat, low-calorie sources of antioxidants and phytochemicals, fiber, nutrients, vitamins, and miner-als, plus they have the hard-core filling power to displace less healthy foods.

Here are some of what I call the Rainbow Food All-Stars:

Rainbow Veggies

- Carrots
- Red and green peppers
- Squash
- Purple cabbage
- Eggplant
- Asparagus
- Beets
- Tomatoes
- Avocados
- Celery
- Cucumber
- Zucchini
- Pumpkin
- Radishes
- Turnips
- Garlic
- Leeks
- Onions
- Corn
- Beans, lentils, and peas
- Tofu, made from soybeans
- Potatoes

Rainbow Fruits

- Oranges
- Peaches
- Cantaloupe
- Grapefruit
- Honeydew melons
- Tangerines
- Apricots
- Bananas
- Red and green grapes
- Kiwifruit
- Cranberries
- Pears
- Dates
- Plums
- Grapes
- Cherries
- Mango
- Pineapples
- Raisins

Note: Some experts, like Dr. Walter Willett of the Harvard School of Public Health, do not include potatoes, America's most popular vegetable, in the same category as other vegetables, because they say that eating potatoes isn't linked with the same health benefits as is eating other produce, that potatoes have a high glycemic index, or GI, and that a high-GI diet can contribute to weight gain.

Other experts argue that potatoes can be part of a varied, healthy plant-based diet, and that GI is not a useful guide to making food choices for nondiabetics.

Personally, in moderation, I think spuds rock!

2. ANTIOXIDANT SUPERSTARS: Antioxidants are vitamins, plant chemicals, or minerals that naturally occur in vegetables, fruits, whole grains, beans, and nuts that help protect your body's cells against damage and oxidative stress that can lead to disease.

They can work fast, too: the AICR reports that "some exciting research results show that within a few weeks of adding more fruits and vegetables to their diets, people who do not smoke have increased blood levels of antioxidants and decreased oxidative damage."

The best source of antioxidants is food, not pills.

Rank	Food item	Serving size
1	Small red bean (dried)	½ cup
2	Wild blueberry	1 cup
3	Red kidney bean (dried)	½ cup
4	Pinto bean	½ cup
5	Blueberry (cultivated)	1 cup
6	Cranberry	1 cup (whole)
7	Artichoke (cooked)	1 cup (hearts)
8	Blackberry	1 cup
9	Prune	½ cup
10	Raspberry	1 cup
11	Strawberry	1 cup
12	Red Delicious apple	1 whole
13	Granny Smith apple	1 whole
14	Pecan	1 ounce
15	Sweet cherry	1 cup
16	Black plum	1 whole
17	Russet potato (cooked)	1 whole
18	Black bean (dried)	½ cup
19	Plum	1 whole
20	Gala apple	1 whole

Source: 2004 study data by Ronald L. Prior, Ph.D., chemist and nutritionist, United States Department of Agriculture's Arkansas Children's Nutrition Center. Antioxidant capacity doesn't necessarily reflect exact health benefit, which depends on how antioxidants are used in the body.

The preceding box is a list of the top twenty foods that a major study ranked highest in total antioxidant capacity per serving size. This is not a ranking of the absolute most nutritious of all foods, but examples of great sources of antioxidants that you should enjoy in your diet.

3. SUPERPOWER GREENS: LEAFY AND CRUCIFEROUS VEGGIES: These two elite categories of gorgeous veggies are credited in some studies as scoring high in extra disease-fighting potential, and include:

- Kale
- Collard greens
- Spinach
- Bok choy
- Swiss chard
- Mustard greens
- Beet greens
- Lettuce
- Turnip greens
- Arugula
- Lemon balm
- Kohlrabi
- Endive
- Escarole
- Broccoli
- Cabbage
- Brussels sprouts
- Cauliflower (OK, they're white, not green!)

I confess to you that I have yet to develop a taste for broccoli. I need to work on that, because it is a spectacular little nutritional powerhouse veggie. Collard greens, on the other hand, I eat every which way I can.

4. WHOLE GRAINS: A source of fiber, nutrients, and good complex carbohydrates, whole grains may have benefits for our heart and immune systems, and may defend against diabetes. Tip: Look for "100 percent whole grain" on the package or ingredient list.

Whole grains include brown rice, oatmeal, barley, bulgur, buckwheat groats (also known as kasha), millet, and quinoa (pronounced "keen-wa").

5. SUPERFISH: These fish are both rich in omega-3 good fats and low in environmental contaminants, according to oceansalive.org: sardines, canned Alaskan salmon, Alaskan cod, Atlantic herring, Atlantic mackerel, and farmed oysters.

6. EXTRA-VIRGIN OLIVE OIL: Olive oil is rich in heart-protective mono-unsaturated fats, which can cut the risk of clogged arteries and lower bad LDL cholesterol while raising good HDL cholesterol. Extra-virgin olive oil is most nutritious. Watch the calories, though: all fat contains 120 calories a tablespoon.

7. CANOLA OIL: Instead of cooking with butter, animal fats, or other methods high in heart-unhealthy saturated fats, choose a plant-based oil like canola, which is low in saturated fat and high in heart-healthy mono-unsaturated fats. Ditto on the calorie caution: fat has 120 calories a table-spoon.

8. NUTS: Choose nutrient-packed unsalted nuts instead of less-healthy snack foods. Almonds and walnuts are great choices, low in bad satu-rated fat and high in good unsaturated fat. Other choices: Brazil nuts, cashew nuts, hazelnuts, macadamia nuts, pecans, pine nuts, pistachios, and peanuts. Tip: Keep your quantities moderate, since nuts are high in calories.

9. SWEET POTATOES: A close relative of the nutritious yam, the sweet potato is the veggie that's in a class by itself because it tastes almost like dessert and it's really nutritious. The Center for Science in the Public Interest has ranked sweet potatoes as the number-one vegetable in nutri-tion. A good source of vitamins A and C, fiber, potassium, and beta-carotene, you can microwave one in minutes. Tip: Eat the potato with the nutritious skin on, and skip the gooey toppings. Sweet potatoes are natu-rally sweet and scrumptious on their own.

10. CUSTOM-BOTTLED PERSONAL ICE WATER: Have you ever had this? It's fantastic. This is my fancy name for tap water you bottle and chill yourself in handy grab-and-go bottles.

The beverage companies will hate me for this, but let's forget sweet-ened soda: it can help make you fat, and it's so last century. Forget diet soda. Who needs it? You absolutely don't need sugared sports drinks, ei-ther, unless you're a hard-core performance athlete. They're a waste of money.

I know that this is a radical, revolutionary, completely bizarre idea for many Americans to digest, given the staggering size and scope of the flavored-beverage industry. But unless you're drinking some of your fruit and veggies fresh (which I will soon suggest you do), *there's absolutely no reason for you to waste money on almost any beverage other than the earth's beautiful gift to us: delicious, crisp, ice-cold water.*

All you need to do is buy a bunch of plastic bottled waters, one time. When you're done, fill those bottles up with tap water, assuming it's safe in your town, like it is where I live, in New York City. Otherwise invest in a water filter, which will quickly pay for itself.

Then stick 'em in a nice cold spot in your home and office refrigerators, grab, and guzzle. It's that simple. Almost totally free. You'll look stylish, because you're showing off a fancy water bottle.

And the earth will love you, because you're helping fix the terrible pollution problem caused by millions of perfectly good and reusable plastic bottles being thrown in the garbage every day.

Living Well Checkoff: Day 2

I'm going to make copies of the Living Well Shopping List below, stick it in my purse, briefcase, or wallet, and use it as a guide to my shopping, to remind me of the types of things I should remember to include and emphasize in my diet.

Check Here: _____

LIVING WELL POWERHOUSE FOODS SHOPPING LIST

DON'T FORGET TO INCLUDE A VARIETY OF THESE FOODS IN YOUR DIET

Make Copies for Your Wallet, Purse, Refrigerator Door

RAINBOW VEGGIES
Kale
Collard greens
Bok choy
Swiss chard
Mustard greens
Beet greens
Lettuce
Turnip greens
Lemon balm
Kohlrabi
Endive
Escarole
Broccoli
Arugula
Cabbage
Brussels sprouts
Cauliflower
Carrots
Red & green peppers
Squash
Purple cabbage
Eggplant
Asparagus
Tomatoes
Avocados
Cucumber
Zucchini
Pumpkin
Radishes
Turnips
Garlic
Leeks
Onions

Corn
Sweet potatoes & yams
Artichoke
Beans, lentils & peas
Small red beans
Pinto beans
Red kidney beans
Black beans
Tofu
Celery*
Potatoes*
Lettuce*
Sweet bell peppers*
Spinach*

RAINBOW FRUITS
Honeydew melons
Tangerines
Apricots
Oranges
Bananas
Red and green grapes
Kiwifruit
Cranberries
Dates
Plums
Blueberries
Blackberries
Raspberries
Strawberries*
Prune
Mango
Pineapples
Raisins

Dates
Peaches*
Nectarines*
Cantaloupe
Apples*
Cherries*
Grapes (imported*)
Pears*

WHOLE GRAINS
Brown rice
Oatmeal
Barley
Bulgur
Buckwheat groats/kasha
Millet
Quinoa

COOKING OIL
Extra-virgin olive oil
Canola oil

SUPERFISH HIGH IN OMEGA-3S/LOW IN MERCURY & PCBS
Sardines
Alaskan salmon
Alaskan cod
Atlantic herring
Atlantic mackerel
Farmed oysters

ADDITIONAL HEALTHY FISH
Abalone (U.S. farmed)
Arctic char (farmed)
Catfish (U.S. farmed)
Caviar (U.S. farmed)
Clams (farmed)
Crab, Dungeness, snow (Canada), stone
Crawfish (U.S.)
Halibut, Pacific (Alaskan)
Mahimahi (U.S. Atlantic)
Mussels (farmed)
Scallops, bay (farmed)
Shrimp, northern (Canada), Oregon pink (U.S. farmed)
Spot prawns
Striped bass (farmed)
Sturgeon (U.S. farmed)
Tilapia (U.S.)

UNSALTED NUTS
Almonds
Walnuts
Brazil nuts
Cashew nuts
Hazelnuts
Macadamia nuts
Pecans
Pine nuts
Pistachios
Peanuts

Don't Forget:
When buying canned veggies and fruit, look for little or no sodium or added sugar.
When buying dairy products, choose low-fat and no-fat versions.
When buying meat and poultry, go for lean cuts and trim off visible fat.

* The Environmental Working Group (EWG) reports that these twelve items have tested highest among produce for pesticides, so the group suggests we buy organic versions of these foods. The EWG's "cleanest 12" list of produce items lowest in pesticides: onions, avocado, sweet corn (frozen), pineapples, mango, sweet peas (frozen), asparagus, kiwi, bananas, cabbage, broccoli, eggplant. Source: www.foodnews.org.

LIVING WELL EXPERT
Barbara J. Rolls, Ph.D.

Dr. Barbara J. Rolls is Helen A. Guthrie chair and professor, department of nutritional sciences at Penn State University.

Dr. Rolls is one of the most widely respected leaders in the field of diet and nutrition, and she has popularized the theory that food "calorie density" affects satiety, or fullness, and body weight. This theory is considered by many researchers to be one of the major keys to weight control and health.

She is the author of the *New York Times* #1 bestseller *The Volumetrics Weight-Control Plan*, which in 2007 was ranked by *Consumer Reports* as the best diet book, with the evidence to back it up.

I firmly believe in what Dr. Rolls has to say. Without knowing it, I've been following the foundations of Dr. Rolls's approach for years now—loading up on healthy, low-calorie-density foods like vegetables, fruits, soups, salads, blended drinks, lean proteins, and whole grains. They are close to a magic bullet for weight control, because they have an extraordinary property, according to Dr. Rolls: they fill you up and help you reach a state of "satiety" superefficiently, and help protect you from overeating.

By the way, I think her idea of "stealth vegetables" is brilliant. You should try it at home with your family!

Most people don't understand that eating for weight management and healthy eating are the same thing.

You want food that is high in nutrient density while being low in calorie density, which simply means "calories per bite" or "calories per gram." You need to look at Nutrition Facts labels.

(continued)

Water-rich foods are great. Water adds weight and volume, and no calories. Water content is the key to giving you satisfying portions of food. With a lower-calorie-density meal, you get so much more food to enjoy.

Fruits and vegetables are absolutely key players. They fill you up very efficiently. They are water-rich, they are full of nutrients, and they have fiber. Just don't drown them in oil and fat.

It seems like every week we are discovering new benefits to fruits and vegetables, but most of us are not getting enough of them. Since we're facing an epidemic of childhood obesity, we conducted an experiment with calorie density and three-to-five-year-old children.

We took a pasta with red sauce and reduced the fat a little. Then we blended in broccoli and cauliflower to increase the vegetable content of the sauce. The kids liked the sauce with the "stealth veggies" just as much as regular sauce, and they wound up eating significantly more veggies.

We also do these tests with adults in our laboratory all the time. We'll reduce calorie density by a third by reducing fat and increasing veggies. People don't notice!

Vegetables may seem more expensive, but they don't have to be. You can get canned vegetables like corn and green beans on sale sometimes for thirty cents a can. That's pretty darn cheap! Canned tomatoes are as good a cheap dish as you can get. You can buy fresh vegetables in season, and you can buy them frozen when they're on sale.

Blended vegetable and fruit drinks are fine, too, although whole fruit and whole veggies may be more filling. You get more satisfaction if you actually sat down and chewed whole fruits and vegetables, on a big plate.

I'm not an advocate of the glycemic index (GI) as an approach for selecting foods. It varies from individual to individual, and it changes when you mix foods together. It's too darn complicated for most people and is not a practical guide to use. I think the calorie-density approach makes much more sense.

For example, the potato fares badly under the glycemic index approach, which is sad. The potato is a notoriously "high GI" food, but it is low in calorie density, and if you put a good topping on it, it makes a good meal.

We need good-quality lean protein. I personally eat quite a bit of lean chicken, tofu, beans, pulses, and fish. And lean beef and pork in moderation—why not?

Focus on the healthier fats. Try to get the saturated animal fats down, and favor the polyunsaturated and monounsaturated fats from things like nuts, avocados, olive oil, and fish. But don't forget that fat has twice as many calories in a given portion as carbohydrate.

For a low-calorie-density breakfast, go for bran cereals. I personally add to my cereal some nonfat milk, nonfat plain yogurt, fruit, and a little sugar. If you like eggs, that's OK, too. If you're worried about total calories, and cholesterol, you can use just the egg white.

People are very optimistic that there is some kind of magic answer. But you need to be aware that if some author is telling you that it's easy, and pounds are going to melt away without exercise and calorie control, then you should be pretty suspicious. It doesn't work like that.

Don't spend money and risk your health on some kind of wacky plan that cuts out huge food groups. We need variety. That's what keeps us going.

(continued)

Tip #1: Look for low-calorie-density food that gives you the fewest calories and the most nutrients per bite, or per gram. That means eat fruits and vegetables, whole grains, salads, legumes like beans and lentils, soups, lean protein, and unprocessed foods.

Tip #2: Eat smaller portions of foods that pack a lot of calories into the portion, such as cookies, crackers, red meat, candy, chips, and butter.

Tip #3: Have a soup, salad, or smoothie as a first course. Our tests have shown that if you have a thick smoothie made of nonfat yogurt, fruit, and ice as a first course of a meal, it can help you eat fewer calories overall. Soups and salads as a first course have the same impact— they help fill you up so you eat less of the main course.

Tip #4: Try using "stealth vegetables." Just tweak the dishes you already enjoy! In a stew, for example, sneak in more vegetables and decrease the proportion of fatty meat. ■

Pour on the Green Drinks

've discovered that there is a secret to healthy eating.

It's what I call the Power of Adding In.

Most diets immediately start telling you what you can't have. Many people get so caught up in the idea of a diet meaning taking things away that they don't really consider what you have to put in to make your body run efficiently.

My Living Well Program is not a diet—it's a way of opening the door to healthy eating and exercise. And blended veggie and fruit drinks are a delicious way to get those rainbow veggies and fruits into your body.

So don't worry about what you're going to take out of your diet; *instead, concentrate on the delicious, nutritionally high-power stuff you're going to enjoy gradually adding in.*

And adding in blended Green Drinks to your life is a great way to begin.

In a perfect world, we would be eating lots of fruits and veggies throughout the day, in their whole and natural forms.

But you and I live in the ultra-busy, time-crazed, running-around world, where we can't always do this. My solution is to turn fruit and vegetables into handy, grab-and-guzzle drinks.

I am flat-out crazy about fresh, natural fruit and vegetable drinks. I chug Green Drinks in the morning when I wake up, in the late morning and at midafternoon for a pick-me-up, and anytime I feel like a blast of cool, sweet, mind-blowing nutrition. I even take them with me in glass jars and a travel pack when I travel!

To me, the feeling I get from Green Drinks is light-years better than coffee, soda, or a candy bar.

What's the secret? I fire them up myself in a blender or juicer at home, so they taste fresh and delicious. I love these drinks a thousand times better than the kind you buy in a bottle or at a juice stand for exactly that reason. No added sugars or powders with who-knows-what in them.

If you're trying to get your child or someone else in your home to start eating more vegetables and fruits, this is a fun way to start.

I just want you to get used to putting this intoxicating, soul-quenching green stuff in your body!

So many people are afraid of vegetables. They'll say, "I can't do it! I hate vegetables! I hate the way they taste! No, no, I'll never be able to do it." Well, heck yeah, you can do it! With Green Drinks as a start, it's easier than you think.

Now these Green Drinks are not substitutes for an overall diet rich in many kinds of fruits and veggies, but they are a tasty, fun, and easy way of easing into one—and a great way of reaching for fruit and veggie power instead of a sugary drink or empty, high-calorie snack.

There are two kinds of Green Drinks—blended drinks (or smoothies), using the whole fruit or veggie, and juice drinks, where the fiber pulp is extracted by a juicer.

For me, both kinds are great since they both include many nutrients, antioxidants, and phytochemicals; but blended drinks are better since the fiber is a big nutritional benefit. About two-thirds of what I drink is blended, one-third is juice. And I often save the pulp from juice drinks and add it to soups.

Living Well Checkoff: Day 3

I'm going to start enjoying some blended drinks, as a way of getting the power of fruits and veggies into my body.

Check Here: _____

MONTEL'S GREEN DRINKS "STARTER" RECIPES

Try one in the morning. Then experiment with different flavors over the next few weeks. They're terrific at whatever time of day you like, but the morning is my favorite time for a Green Drink because it gives me a blast of nutrition and energy that helps power me through the day.

On Sunday afternoon you can go to the grocery store, buy your vegetables and fruits, go home and whip up three or four bottles of Green Drinks and toss them in the refrigerator until you're ready to have them. You're all set for the next two or three days.

These drinks only take a few minutes to make—give them a try! You do need a blender (Vita-Mix is best) and a juicer, but they're very worthwhile investments.

Sweet 'n Easy Green Smoothie

This is a healthful, delightful drink with a perky pale green color. The kids will love it!

MAKES 2–4 SERVINGS.

Ingredients
> 2 bananas, peeled
> 3 oranges, peeled and quartered
> 1 head of romaine lettuce
> 4 cups of cold water

Procedure
> In a Vita-Mix blender, add ingredients in order: bananas, oranges, and then romaine. Add water to the "Max Fill" line on the blender. Blend all ingredients at medium, then high speed until smooth. Serve chilled. Will keep for 2–3 days in refrigeration.

Advanced Version: Over time, experiment with introducing new ingredients like these to the drink:

- Parsley
- Collards
- Celery
- Cilantro
- Green and red leaf lettuce
- Kale
- Bok choy
- Swiss chard
- Red beet
- Mango
- Seedless grapes
- Cucumber
- Carrot
- Green apples

Tropical Fruit Smoothie

Wonderfully colorful, creamy, and delicious, this smoothie is pure pleasure.

MAKES 1–2 SERVINGS.

Ingredients
1 mango, peeled and seeded
1 papaya, peeled and seeded
1 banana, peeled
1 orange, peeled
5 cubes ice

Procedure
In a Vita-Mix blender, process ingredients until smooth. Enjoy immediately, or keep 2–3 days in refrigeration.

Triple C Juice

Triple C stands for carrots, celery, and cucumber. This delicious combination is great on its own, or as a base for your further Green Drink experimentation. Try adding leafy green vegetables, such as collards, kale, chard, lettuce, and bok choy as desired. You can save the extracted pulp, which is rich in healthy fiber—refrigerate right away and save for up to 1 day to add to soups as a thickener, or to meat loaf, a casserole, or vinaigrette as a flavor booster.

MAKES 1–2 SERVINGS.

Ingredients

3 large carrots

3 celery stalks

3 cucumbers

Procedure

Pass all ingredients through a juicer and serve immediately. Will also keep 2–3 days in refrigeration.

All-Green Juice

For the more adventurous, green vegetables and green fruits combine to create a flavorful and nutritious green juice.

MAKES 1–2 SERVINGS.

Ingredients

    2 cucumbers

    2 celery stalks

    2 green chard leaves

    2 kale leaves

    2 green apples

    2 small limes, peeled

Procedure

Pass all ingredients through juicer and serve immediately. Will also keep 2–3 days in refrigeration. The extracted pulp can be refrigerated right away for up to 1 day to add to soups as a thickener or to meat loaf, a casserole, or vinaigrette as a flavor booster.

Another thing I like to do with pulp is put it in a bowl, add a little water just hot enough to make it blend together, and then let it cool down and eat it like cold Italian soup. You can fire up a bowl for a quick breakfast, and you're out the door!

LIVING WELL EXPERT
David Grotto, R.D.

David Grotto, R.D., is a registered dietitian and spokesperson for the American Dietetic Association (ADA). With more than sixty-seven thousand members, the ADA is the largest organization of food and nutrition professionals in the United States.

Registered dietitians are often the unsung heroes of nutrition. These guys know more about nutrition than a great many doctors.

Absolutely anyone can call themselves a nutritionist, so you've got to watch out for a lot of bogus credentials out there. But a registered dietitian is by definition someone with an advanced degree from an accredited school, who must pass professional certification. Check to see if your nutritionist also has the "R.D." credential. If they do, it's a good sign.

David Grotto is a man after my own heart. He is a leading nutritional expert who applies the lessons of healthy eating at home with his own family, and he does it by making food fun, delicious, and enjoyable. One of his tactics is my favorite, too: blended drinks.

This is a hugely important point—healthy eating should not be a chore: it can be a treat and a joy, and it must be made a natural part of a family's life.

I'll speak to you not only as spokesperson for the American Dietetic Association but also as a father of three daughters. I have an eight-year-old, a ten-year-old, and a thirteen-year-old.

In my home, a blended fruit and vegetable drink can quite often be the base of a meal.

(continued)

When you've got picky kids at home and whatever you want to serve just doesn't seem to resonate or strike a chord with them, a shake or a smoothie should go over very well, as it does in my home. Sometimes the good stuff has to be disguised to be added to the diet. A smoothie is a great base to add in some things that your kids won't even notice are there.

Take, for example, whey protein. It's an excellent source of protein, ranking near the top of what's called the protein efficiency ratio.

My oldest daughter announced to us two years ago that she wants to become a vegetarian, and I was concerned that she get enough protein. So I started making smoothies for the family that included whey and a variety of different fruits, and I even snuck in some vegetables. And they were none the wiser!

We're not full-disclosure about everything we do with our kids!

When you juice produce and extract the pulp, you are deriving limited benefits from that fruit or vegetable. You get some benefits, but they're limited. The research is very clear that Americans need at least twenty-five to thirty-five grams of fiber per day, and getting in whole produce with the pulp and fiber is a way to help accomplish that. So a blended drink is better than a pulp-extracted juice.

It's about changing the mind-set, too.

It's OK for kids to think a blended produce drink is a treat. It's every bit as nutritious as picking fruit off the vine or vegetables out of the garden. There's no discernible difference in fiber, phytochemicals, or any other benefits between blending produce in a blender or a food processor versus chopping it up and putting it in a pan.

It's all good! ■

Unleash the Raw Strength of Salads

Enjoying food should be a multisensory experience: a symphony not only of tastes but of textures, smells, and magnificent colors.

And nothing quite tantalizes the senses like a rich, powerful salad.

If you're eating a typical American diet, you should start bringing more salads into your life—as of today, Day 4 of the Living Well Program.

By the way, when I say "salad," I don't mean some people's idea of the standard American salad: a few anemic, elderly iceberg lettuce leaves parked next to a limp, cold, long-dead tomato on a little dish.

That's not a salad!

I'm talking about off-the-hook, hard-rocking power salads that make your taste buds moan and cry out for Mama. Salads that fill you up and deliver deep satisfaction, with a soul-refreshing blizzard of phytochemicals, antioxidants, fiber, vitamins, and minerals.

You can call me crispy-crunchy, but that's OK with me. I think salads are the earth's gift to us, and Nature's way of saying, "I love you—now eat!"

Salads are a staple of my diet. They feel like pure life force when you chew them up and gobble them down. I'll have them on their own or I'll add a piece of fish or lean meat to them.

I build a salad like van Gogh painted a picture. I want the brightest, most dazzling colors in there—lots of them.

When I'm on the road and eating at a restaurant, I'll often ask the waiters if they can just chop up and serve me a big bowl filled with a bunch of the freshest multicolor veggies they have. I've tried this in many restaurants, and you'd be surprised how many will do it.

I ask the restaurant for whatever they've got that's *most fresh*: green stuff, purple stuff, red and yellow peppers, avocado, and some walnuts for crunchiness. Toss in some fresh fruit while you're at it: some orange or apple slices. Why not?

Salads are a great way of enjoying the benefits of the Living Well Code, and a great way of getting fresh raw vegetables into your diet.

A recent study of over seventeen thousand adult Americans found that salad consumers had higher intakes of a variety of nutrients, including vitamins C and E, lycopene, folic acid, and alpha- and beta-carotene. The study concluded, "Salad, salad dressing, and raw vegetable consumption can be an effective strategy for enhancing nutritional adequacy and increasing vegetable consumption in the population at large."

Notice that they included salad dressing on the list. That's interesting, since one recent study suggested that a little fat on a salad in the form of dressing or avocado (which is high in monounsaturated good fat) actually helps the body absorb nutrients better, versus no dressing or no-fat dressing.

Salads may even help us with weight control, according to a laboratory study conducted by Professor Barbara Rolls and her colleagues at the department of nutritional sciences at Penn State University.

They found that having a first course of a big (300-gram) salad with a relatively low amount of calories from dressing and cheese increased the feeling of fullness, and reduced the total amount of calories eaten at the meal by 12 percent overall, versus a meal eaten with no first course.

So starting today, I want you to start eating more salads. Make them big, make them colorful, and make them often.

I'm going to start enjoying bigger, more healthy salads, as a first course and even as a main course. I'll hold off on the extra salt and excessive high-calorie creamy dressings.

Check Here: _____

MONTEL'S THREE FAVORITE POWER SALAD RECIPES

Strong-to-the-Finish Spinach Salad with Warm Balsamic Apple Vinaigrette

Fresh spinach has strong crunchy leaves. The warm vinaigrette gently softens the spinach and adds a sweet sting to this salad.

SERVES 4–6.

Ingredients

$\frac{1}{2}$ pint cherry tomatoes, halved

$\frac{1}{2}$ red onion, thinly sliced

2 tablespoons raw shelled walnuts, crumbled

6 ounces fresh spinach leaves

3 tablespoons extra-virgin olive oil

1 tablespoon balsamic vinegar

$\frac{1}{2}$ teaspoon salt

freshly ground black pepper to taste

1 red apple

Procedure

In a large salad bowl, combine tomatoes, onion slices, walnuts, and spinach. Set aside. In a small mixing bowl, whisk together oil and vinegar. Add salt and pepper. Warm oil and vinegar mixture in a small saucepan over very low heat. While vinaigrette is warming (about 1–2 minutes), cut apple into quarters and remove core and seeds. Cut apple into thin bite-sized slices. Add apple slices to vinaigrette and mix thoroughly. Remove warm vinaigrette from heat and pour over salad. Toss, serve, and enjoy.

Southwestern Macho-Man Salad

Who said salads have to be dainty and delicate? Featuring hot peppers and raw garlic, this salad is not for the faint of heart. It is, however, so easily made that even the most machismo will still feel manly whipping one up. Try experimenting with different hot peppers (habanero, serrano, cherry pepper) and chili powders (cayenne, chipotle, ancho) to make this salad your own.

SERVES 4–6.

Ingredients

3 romaine lettuce hearts

4 ears of corn, shucked and kernels sliced off

1 red pepper, cut into large chunks

1 yellow pepper, cut into large chunks

1 jalapeño pepper, sliced into rounds

1 clove raw garlic, minced

2 avocados, peel and pit removed, cubed

2 tablespoons extra-virgin olive oil

1 tablespoon fresh squeezed lemon juice (approx. 2 lemons)

1 tablespoon raw honey or agave nectar

1 teaspoon chili powder

½ teaspoon salt

freshly ground black pepper to taste

Garnish

1 tablespoon raw pumpkin seeds

¼ head fresh cilantro, stemmed, finely chopped

Procedure

In a large salad bowl, tear romaine hearts into bite-sized pieces. Add corn, peppers, garlic, avocados, oil, lemon juice, honey or agave, chili powder, salt, and pepper. Toss thoroughly and divide into bowls. Garnish each bowl of salad with raw pumpkin seeds and fresh cilantro. Serve and enjoy.

Kalamata Olive and Kale Salad with Creamy Almond Butter Dressing

Kale is a dark leafy green with very high nutritional value. It comes in a few different varieties. Most common are green kale (curly kale), red kale, and dinosaur kale (lacinato kale). I prefer green curly kale for this salad. Most people turn up their noses at eating kale raw. But once they try it, they usually come back for more.

When you combine all these ingredients, the result is amazing; it's like you're eating a piece of the finest meat. Incredible sensations will blossom in your mouth.

MAKES 4–6 SERVINGS.

Ingredients

2 large heads kale, stemmed and cut into bite-sized pieces

½ cup kalamata pitted olives, sliced into rounds

1 small red onion, halved and sliced thin

1 carrot, grated

4 tablespoons raw almond butter (toasted almond butter is OK if raw is unavailable)

juice of 2 lemons

1–2 tablespoons agave nectar to taste

1 tablespoon slivered almonds

1 tablespoon chopped parsley

freshly ground black pepper to taste

Procedure

In a large salad bowl, toss together kale, olives, onion slices, and grated carrot. In a small mixing bowl, whisk together almond butter, lemon juice, and agave to make creamy almond butter dressing. Toss salad with dressing. Garnish with slivered almonds and chopped parsley. Sprinkle with black pepper and serve.

LIVING WELL EXPERT
Karen Collins, R.D.

Karen Collins, R.D., is nutrition adviser for the American Institute for Cancer Research (AICR). She is a registered dietitian and an authority on the connections between diet, exercise, lifestyle, and cancer.

In late 2007, the AICR published a landmark expert report, "Food, Nutrition, Physical Activity and the Prevention of Cancer," which is the most comprehensive scientific assessment of the links between diet and cancer ever conducted.

Over the years I've heard a lot of anecdotal information and stories about the connections between diet and cancer. They're interesting, but they're not science. That's why it's great to hear a top expert like Karen Collins tackle this absolutely crucial subject.

According to Collins and the AICR, this is a "fantastic news" story: your food choices and lifestyle can have a major positive impact on lowering your risk for key forms of cancer.

I am really impressed by the AICR's idea of "the New American Plate," which calls for simple "tweaks" in our normal eating patterns that can transform our diets into potent cancer-fighting weapons.

Healthy eating is one of the best tools to help lower your risk of cancer. People don't fully understand this at all.

What we eat affects virtually every stage of cancer development: the initial damage to the DNA that starts the cancer process, cell growth and reproduction, and the ability of cancer cells to grow and spread.

Healthy eating alone certainly can't totally protect you from cancer, but it's one of our most potent weapons, along with avoiding tobacco.

At the American Institute for Cancer Research we developed what we call the New American Plate as a simple picture of how to put a cancer-prevention diet into practice. It's based on two ideas: adjusting the proportions of what we eat and adjusting the portions of what we eat.

It's a very simple shift.

The goal of the New American Plate is moving toward a more plant-based diet. It doesn't mean you have to totally give up meat, or become a vegetarian. The formula is very simple: at least two-thirds of your plate should be things like vegetables, fruits, whole grains, beans, and nuts. Whole grains are also a good choice for cancer protection.

If you're going to have a turkey sandwich for lunch, have it on whole-grain bread. Instead of rounding it out with potato chips or cookies, round it out with some fruit or salad or vegetable or a soup. For dinner, just flip-flop the proportions so the meat portion is smaller. The recommendation is to eat no more than three ounces of red meat a day, which is about the size of a deck of cards.

There are a number of ways that fruits and vegetables are involved in cancer prevention.

Initially, they were looked at primarily as the sources of vitamins

(continued)

and minerals that were linked with lower cancer risk, like vitamin C, vitamin A, and beta-carotene. But we now realize that there are thousands of natural compounds called phytochemicals in fruits and vegetables that probably have an even larger impact on cancer prevention. They act throughout the cancer process.

Many of them are antioxidants. What antioxidants do is neutralize compounds called free radicals that damage the DNA in our cells and begin changing them into cancer cells. Some phytochemicals also stimulate enzymes that can actually deactivate or "switch off" carcinogens.

When you look at parts of the world that have less cancer, like the Mediterranean or China and Japan, you might say their diets are nothing like each other. But there is a common thread: they are plant-based diets.

Variety is a huge factor. Rather than loading up on a few "powerhouse" fruits and vegetables, go for a wide variety. There is research suggesting that people who concentrate on variety enjoy greater DNA protection.

People often don't think outside the box with vegetables. They think they're too much work, or don't taste good. I sympathize; I grew up with vegetables being overcooked, mushy, and not flavored well. But here are some tips:

1. Go the AICR.org Web site, punch in almost any fruit or vegetable, and you'll come up with some great ways to fix and enjoy it.
2. To add flavor to vegetables, use lemon juice, spices, herbs, onion, or garlic.
3. Frozen produce is a great time-saver. It's already been washed and chopped; just stick it in the microwave or in the steamer.
4. Use canned beans; they're all cooked and ready to go. Just put them in a strainer to drain and rinse off the high-sodium liquid in the can.

5. Try new vegetables you haven't had before. Add a new vegetable to a dish you like already, like a casserole, a stew, or a stir-fry.

Fresh and frozen are pretty much equal. Certainly, fresh ingredients from your garden are going to be the highest in nutrients. But frozen is going to be just as good as fresh for most people. Either is excellent. Canning produce may somewhat reduce heat-sensitive nutrients like vitamin C, but it may increase the availability of good things like beta-carotene in carrots and lycopene in tomatoes.

The minimum recommended amount for health is five servings of fruits and vegetables a day, with seven to ten being optimal. That's easier to achieve than most people realize, because a serving is only a half a cup or a cup, depending on the type of produce. It's easy if you make produce a part of your meals all day long.

If one of those seven to ten servings is a 100 percent fruit or vegetable juice, that's great. It's convenient and enjoyable. But it's not quite equal to the whole fruit because first it's not going to be as high in fiber. Second, when you squeeze the juice you're often not using the skin, and many phytochemicals are concentrated in outer areas of the plant.

The most important thing is simply to eat more fruits and vegetables, in a wide variety.

But we're living in a society where huge portions are everywhere, so you need to pay attention not only to what you eat but to how much you eat.

It doesn't mean you should go hungry, but there is a lot of research that shows that the more food is in front of you, the more you'll eat, just because it's there. Weight control is very important for lowering the risk of a number of cancers, and physical activity is, too. ■

Fire Up the Power of Fish

I **have a love affair with fish.**

It's one of my favorite comfort foods.

I eat fish the way some people eat meat. I have it at home at any hour of the day, and I order it on the road, in restaurants and hotels.

Give me a beautiful, gently cooked piece of succulent whitefish drizzled with a little miso sauce, lemon, and fresh herbs—and I'm in food heaven.

Fish occupies an exalted position in the Living Well Code, and rightly so.

Fish is a lean, delicious source of protein and other nutrients that is relatively low in saturated fat, and according to nutritional researchers, certain species of fish may help protect our hearts.

Omega-3 fatty acids have received a tidal wave of good press in recent years for their probable heart-protective effects, and several fish species are considered among the best, most efficient sources of them. Omega-3 fatty acids are also available in some vegetable oils, like linseed, flaxseed, walnut, and canola, but they may not be quite as beneficial as those found in fish.

In 2002, the World Health Organization found that "most, but not all, population studies have shown that fish consumption is associated with a reduced risk of coronary heart disease."

In 2005, the U.S. government's Dietary Guidelines for Americans, based on hundreds of research studies, declared: "A reduced risk of both sudden death and CHD [coronary heart disease] death in adults is associated with the consumption of two servings (approx. 8 oz.) per week of fish high in the n-3 fatty acids [omega-3s] called eicosapentaenoic acid (EPA) and docosahexaenoic acid (DHA). To benefit from the potential cardioprotective effects of EPA and DHA, the weekly consumption of two servings of fish, particularly fish rich in EPA and DHA, is suggested."

Omega-3s from fish are not only being studied for their possible ability to protect against cardiac arrhythmias and sudden cardiac death, but also for potential benefits in fighting depression, dementia, and inflammatory conditions like arthritis.

The key to eating fish the healthy Living Well way is to eat it baked, poached, or broiled or straight out of the can—not battered or fried.

There are, however, real problems with *some* fish: certain species may have high amounts of mercury, or may contain PCBs (polychlorinated biphenyls, which are toxic industrial compounds), or dioxins or pesticides. Also, some fish are harvested in ways that environmental groups consider ecologically irresponsible.

The Food and Drug Administration (FDA) and the Environmental Protection Agency (EPA) have issued warnings for women who may become pregnant, pregnant women, nursing mothers, and young children *not to eat shark, swordfish, king mackerel, or tilefish* because they contain high levels of mercury. The FDA and EPA recommend these groups eat up to 12 ounces (two average meals) a week of a variety of fish and shellfish that are lower in mercury.

Now here's the fantastic news.

You absolutely don't have to avoid fish altogether. That, in my opinion, would be tragic, because you'd be missing out on a superior source of nutrition.

And you don't have to go crazy trying to figure out on your own which fish are "good" and which fish are "bad." Much of the homework has already been done for you by several leading environmental groups, including one called Oceans Alive, which publishes a great rundown on fish on their Web site, oceansalive.org.

MONTEL'S GOOD FISH LISTS

SuperFish: These top-notch fish, which I call SuperFish, have a triple health punch, according to oceansalive.org—they're rich in heart-healthy omega-3 fatty acids, they're low in environmental contaminants like mercury and PCBs, and they're harvested in an environmentally responsible way. If the world of fish was a health and beauty contest, these babies would be in the winners' circle.

- Anchovies
- Herring—Atlantic (United States, Canada)
- Mackerel—Atlantic
- Oysters (farmed)
- Sablefish/black cod (Alaskan)
- Sardines
- Salmon—wild (Alaskan); canned pink or sockeye (Alaskan)

Living Well Tip: Canned Alaskan salmon is a superconvenient choice, and the skin and bones in some versions are completely edible and extranutritious. Try using salmon the way you used to use tuna, in sandwiches, for example.

Farmed Atlantic salmon, which sounds tasty, has the risk of high levels of PCB contaminants, according to oceansalive.org. Alaskan salmon looks like a better choice.

Additional Healthy Fish: These fish choices, while not high in omega-3s, are still hailed by oceansalive.org as both low in environmental contaminants and harvested in an environmentally responsible manner.

- Abalone (U.S. farmed)
- Arctic char (farmed)
- Catfish (U.S. farmed)
- Caviar (U.S. farmed)
- Clams (farmed)
- Crab—Dungeness, snow (Canada), stone
- Crawfish (U.S.)
- Halibut—Pacific (Alaskan)
- Mahimahi (U.S. Atlantic)
- Mussels (farmed)
- Scallops—bay (farmed)
- Shrimp—northern (Canada), Oregon pink (U.S. farmed)
- Spot prawns
- Striped bass (farmed)
- Sturgeon (U.S. farmed)
- Tilapia (U.S.)

A Note on Tuna: Albacore ("white") tuna has more mercury than "canned light" tuna, so personally, I avoid albacore and go for "canned light" tuna. It's usually made from skipjack tuna, which, according to oceansalive.org, has contaminant levels that are so low that they do not warrant a consumption advisory.

Check the oceansalive.org Web site for other healthy fish choices.

Living Well Checkoff: Day 5

I'm going to bring more fish from the lists above into my diet, especially fish rich in omega-3s.

Check Here: _____

LIVING WELL FISH RECIPES

Red Miso Soup
with Poached Wild Alaskan Salmon

Variety is the spice of life, and this is a fantastic recipe inspired loosely by the traditional Japanese style of having miso soup and fish, even for breakfast.

That's right, breakfast! Why not? I sometimes enjoy this rich and mellow energy booster as my first meal of the day with a piece of whitefish instead of salmon.

You can enjoy this as a power lunch or in a healthy dinner, too. The dark color and heartiness of red miso combines beautifully with the earthiness of mushrooms and the rich texture of wild salmon.

SERVES 2–3.

Ingredients

4 cups water

½ pound wild Alaskan salmon, skin removed

4 mushrooms, thinly sliced

2 teaspoons low-sodium soy sauce

4 tablespoons red miso paste (adjust to taste)

⅛ teaspoon toasted sesame oil

1 handful baby spinach leaves

2 stalks green onion, sliced into thin rounds

Procedure

In a small pot, bring water to a boil over high heat. While water boils, slice salmon into bite-sized pieces and set aside. Once water boils, bring to a simmer over medium heat. Add salmon to simmering water and cook thoroughly (1–2 minutes) while bringing water back up to a simmer. Remove pot from flame and stir in mushrooms, soy sauce, miso paste, and sesame oil. Ladle soup into bowls and garnish with a few spinach leaves and a generous helping of green onion. Enjoy.

Note: Some miso soup paste can be really high in sodium, so keep an eye on the total sodium count of the miso you use and adjust the amount accordingly.

You can also experiment with yellow and white miso pastes, which generally have less sodium.

Spicy Baked Fish with Herbs

This recipe is from the highly acclaimed DASH Diet developed by the National Heart, Lung and Blood Institute, a department of the National Institutes of Health. DASH stands for Dietary Approaches to Stop Hypertension.

SERVES 4.

Ingredients

Cooking oil spray
1 pound salmon (or other fish) fillet
1 tablespoon extra-virgin olive oil
1 teaspoon spicy seasoning, salt-free
herbs of your choice

Procedure

Preheat oven to 350°F. Spray a casserole dish with cooking oil spray. Wash and dry fish. Place in dish. Mix oil and seasoning and drizzle over fish. Bake uncovered for 15 minutes or until fish flakes with fork. Garnish with fresh herbs. Cut into 4 pieces. Serve with rice.

LIVING WELL EXPERT
Robert Eckel, M.D.

Dr. Robert Eckel is professor of medicine, physiology, and biophysics, and the Charles A. Boettcher II chair in atherosclerosis at the University of Colorado at Denver Health Sciences Center.

In 2005–6 he was president of the American Heart Association (AHA), and was involved in the development of the AHA's acclaimed book *No-Fad Diet: A Personal Plan for Healthy Weight Loss*. He is a leading expert in the areas of nutrition, obesity, metabolism, and diabetes.

I really appreciate how Dr. Eckel points out what we don't know yet about nutrition, and how much of it remains a mystery. But at the same time, he has excellent, concrete suggestions for us to consider, suggestions based strongly on scientific evidence.

According to the AHA, cardiovascular disease is the leading U.S. health problem, and the leading cause of death. At least 58.8 million people in the United States suffer from some form of heart disease. One person in four suffers from some form of cardiovascular disease, including high blood pressure, coronary heart disease, stroke, rheumatic heart disease/rheumatic fever, congenital cardiovascular defects, and congestive heart failure. Almost two out of every five deaths is from cardiovascular disease, and over twenty-six hundred deaths occur each day from cardiovascular disease.

The AHA says that although a strong family history of heart disease and increasing age are heart disease risk factors you can't change, you can take control of a host of other risk factors established by landmark population studies like the Framingham Heart Study. These include high blood cholesterol, high blood pressure, smoking, dietary factors (particularly dietary cholesterol, fat, and sodium), obesity, and physical inactivity.

Some of the best strategies for living well are to prevent excess body fat or get lean, stay fit for your entire life, and improve the quality of your overall "nutritional package."

We've got to develop a basic understanding that losing weight means burning off more calories than you take in. Keeping weight off over the long term is more difficult. There are important differences between losing weight and keeping it off. For the active weight-loss phase, I tend to put the emphasis on eating less. For maintaining weight reduction, you also need a high level of physical activity.

Nutrition research is a different challenge from doing research on a new pharmaceutical. With a drug, you typically have a placebo group, and participants are preferably selected and randomized. We have an outcome that we can trust. But modifying and studying a dietary pattern for decades in a population is impossible to do. So the nutrition science we do have is limited to relatively short-term studies, with end points such as heart attacks, stroke, cancer, and death really inadequately assessed.

We do, however, have a reasonably strong amount of observational data that examines dietary and disease patterns of different populations. These are observational studies, not interventional. The bottom line is that fruits and vegetables, whole grains, fiber, lean poultry, and fish are all things that relate to reduced incidence of heart disease, stroke, diabetes, and cancer, and probably have a benefit on all-cause mortality.

Getting more people to eat a diet that includes these constituents makes a lot of scientific sense. The benefits may go beyond simple

(continued)

biomarker assessments. We can measure cholesterol, we can measure blood pressure, and we can measure glucose tolerance, all of which are favorably modified by a scientifically based healthy diet. But some of the benefits, like reduced risk for heart attack and stroke, are not explained by all of the biomarkers we measure.

In a sense, it's the mystery of good nutrition. There's something good about a healthy diet that can't be quantified in blood, or urine, or other clinical tests. The whole-diet approach appears to create positive outcomes that go beyond our ability to measure all of the individual parts.

People want to take supplements. They want a magic bullet to feel better or live longer. But the evidence for supplements just isn't there, except for rare situations like folic acid for pregnant women to protect their child from neural tube defects. For heart disease, we don't have any hint that there is a benefit from supplements.

So, instead of taking supplements, why don't we eat an overall dietary pattern that has been proven to be beneficial?

Don't be swayed by what your neighbor is doing, or by what the latest *National Enquirer* article may say about a dietary program. Go to credible sources of information like the U.S. Department of Agriculture Nutrition Guidelines, and look at the recommendations put forth by credible professional organizations, such as the American Heart Association and the American Dietetic Association. And don't ignore physical activity as part of a healthy lifestyle. ■

Tap the Energy
of Whole Grains

O ne of the first things I did when I chose to start really Living Well was to pull most of the refined grains out of my diet.

I mostly stopped eating white bread, white pasta, white rice, bagels, and refined cereals, all of which are processed foods, where important nutritional components have been stripped out.

In their place, I cranked up the whole grains, in the form of foods like whole-grain bread, whole-grain cereals, and raw granola made from whole grains, nuts, and fruit.

Now, maybe this is scientific or maybe it's psychosomatic—but as soon as I did this, I felt leaner and had more energy. And I didn't feel the swings of high blood sugar followed by crashes of sleepiness and lethargy I used to feel, for example, after scarfing down a plain white bagel.

Let me tell you, whole grains not only taste richer, chewier, and heartier, they offer an excellent boost for your and your family's health.

Starting today, Day 6 of the Living Well Program, let's welcome whole grains into your daily food life.

One of the really boneheaded consequences of the Atkins craze was the demonization of carbohydrates. "No carb" and "low-carb" became cultural mantras for losing weight. This is ridiculous, because carbohydrates are a crucial source of energy for our brains and bodies as part of an overall healthy diet.

OK, it turns out that Atkins-inspired "anti-carb" cliché was half right: *refined* carbohydrates from foods like highly refined grains are the ones you want to minimize, since essential nutrients have been reduced or removed. But *good, healthy carbohydrates* like whole grains are an essential part of a dietary pattern for Living Well.

A whole grain is, well, literally the whole grain, including the three main parts: the germ, the bran, and the endosperm. By contrast, "refined grains" means the germ and bran have been stripped out during processing. The problem with this is that the bran is what contains the healthy fiber, and the germ is where you'll find most of the nutrients.

It's time to fall in love with whole grains, by making them a cornerstone of your Living Well dietary approach.

7 Reasons to Fall in Love . . . with Whole Grains

1. Whole grains may help protect against cardiovascular disease, type 2 diabetes, and obesity.
2. Whole grains contain healthy fiber, as much as four times more than refined grains.
3. Whole grains are a good source of protein, vitamins, and minerals.
4. Whole grains contain healthy phytochemicals.
5. Whole grains contain healthy antioxidants.
6. Whole grains can help you feel full faster, so you'll eat fewer calories.
7. Emerging research suggests that fiber from whole grains is associated with a lower risk of colorectal cancer.

Today, on average, Americans eat less than one serving of whole grains per day. But the U.S. Dietary Guidelines suggest we eat at least three servings (about equal to three ounces) of whole grains per day, to help reduce the risk of diabetes and heart disease and to help with weight maintenance—preferably by substituting whole grains for re-fined grains.

It's easier to eat those three servings a day than you may think: one slice of bread, one-half cup of cooked rice or pasta, and one cup of break-fast cereal are each equal to about one serving.

Montel's Top Tips for Cranking Up the Whole Grains

- On the ingredient list or package, look for "100 percent whole grain."
- "Whole grain" or "made with whole grain" on the package isn't enough, since such foods may be only partially made from whole grains. In fact, foods labeled with the words "multigrain," "stone-ground," "100 percent wheat," "cracked wheat," "seven-grain," or "bran" are often not whole-grain products.
- Look for the whole grain to be the first ingredient listed in the ingredients list on the food package.
- In general, at least half the grains you consume should come from whole grains, according to the Food and Drug Administration.
- According to the Whole Grains Council, the following, when consumed in a form including the bran, germ, and endosperm, are examples of whole-grain foods and flours:
  - Amaranth
  - Barley
  - Buckwheat
  - Buckwheat groats (also known as kasha)
  - Corn, including whole cornmeal and popcorn
  - Millet
  - Oats, including oatmeal
  - Quinoa
  - Rice, both brown rice and colored rice
  - Rye
  - Sorghum (also called milo)
  - Teff

- Triticale
- Wheat, including varieties such as spelt, emmer, farro, einkorn, Kamut, durum, and forms such as bulgur, cracked wheat, and wheat berries
- Wild rice

Two Quick Whole-Grain Shortcuts

- **90-Second Brown Rice Microwaveable Pouches:** These are a new, superconvenient (although pricier) option. Tip: Skip the high-sodium flavored varieties and buy the plain kind, and then spice it up yourself with herbs or no-sodium seasonings. Eating more brown rice instead of the white stuff you probably grew up on is a great way to get your whole grains. White rice is basically brown rice stripped of its bran and germ, and a lot of good stuff gets lost in the bargain: brown rice has almost ten times as much phosphorus and potassium as white rice, for instance.
- **Instant Oatmeal:** Oatmeal is a filling, low-calorie-density breakfast superstar, boasting soluble fiber that can lower cholesterol in the blood and may help maintain healthy blood pressure and stable insulin and blood sugar levels. Check nutrition labels to buy with minimum sodium and no added sugar, then sweeten with natural fruit, like berries.

LIVING WELL CHECKOFF: DAY 6

I'm going to gradually start eating more whole grains in my diet as a healthier alternative to refined grains.

Check Here: _____

LIVING WELL WHOLE-GRAINS RECIPES

Stir-Fried Chicken with Bok Choy and Steamed Brown Rice

Here's a healthy stir-fry with a whole-grain punch in the form of brown rice.

Set the rice up to cook before you prep the stir-fry and everything will be ready at the same time. Bok choy is best barely cooked, crunchy and delicious. If you can't find it, try substituting fresh celery.

SERVES 4.

BROWN RICE

Ingredients

> 1 cup brown rice
> 1 cup frozen peas, thawed
> ½ teaspoon salt

Procedure

Cook 1 cup of brown rice according to the instructions on the package. When the rice is ready, stir in peas and salt to taste.

STIR-FRIED CHICKEN WITH BOK CHOY

Ingredients

> 2 tablespoons canola oil
> 1 clove garlic, minced
> 1 pound boneless skinless chicken breasts, cut into ¼-inch slices
> 1 large onion, halved, thinly sliced
> 1 bunch bok choy, sliced on the bias
> 1 teaspoon grated ginger
> 1 tablespoon low-sodium soy sauce

Procedure

In a large skillet, heat half of the oil over high heat until very hot. Be sure not to let the oil smoke. Add the garlic, stir, and immediately add the chicken. Stir-fry 1–2 minutes until chicken is partially cooked. Add the remaining oil. Add the onion and stir-fry until ingredients start to brown. Add the bok choy, ginger, and soy sauce. Stir-fry briefly, less than 1 minute, and serve over rice.

Quinoa Stew

I am on a personal crusade to get people to try whole-grain quinoa. Many people haven't even heard of it yet. It's kind of like brown rice, but it's softer and smaller, with a gentle, lightly nutty taste. What's so cool about quinoa is that it's a whole grain, which means it's healthy, and it has a striking ability to pick up the flavors of what you serve it with, almost like tofu does.

Quinoa is delicious when prepared correctly. This requires a prudent washing and gentle toasting of the grains before adding them to boiling water. This takes any inherent bitterness out of the grain and brings forth its natural nutlike qualities.

SERVES 4.

QUINOA

Ingredients

water as needed

1 cup quinoa

Procedure

In a small stock pot, bring 2 cups of water to a boil. Meanwhile, fill a medium mixing bowl with water, thoroughly submerge 1 cup of quinoa, and then strain with a fine-mesh strainer. Repeat 3 times using fresh, clean water each time.

In a large skillet, gently toast the washed and strained quinoa over a low flame, stirring occasionally until the nutty smell of the grain is detected and it has darkened slightly. This may take up to 10 minutes. If the grains are popping, the heat is too high.

Once quinoa is lightly toasted, add to boiling water and reduce to a simmer. Cook 10–15 minutes until all water is absorbed and the round grains sprout tiny little "tails." Strain off any extra cooking liquid and set aside.

STEW

Ingredients

2 large sweet onions, halved, cut into large dices

2 tablespoons extra-virgin olive oil

1 clove garlic, minced

½ pound button mushrooms, cleaned, stems removed, quartered

3 large tomatoes, halved, cut into large dices

1 teaspoon celery seeds

½ teaspoon ground basil

½ teaspoon ground oregano

½ cup water

1 pound carrots, cut into large dices

prepared quinoa

water as needed

¼ pound fresh spinach

Procedure

In a small stock pot, sauté onions in oil over medium heat until translucent (5–10 minutes). Add garlic and mushrooms. Sauté until liquid is released.

Add tomatoes, celery seeds, basil, oregano, and water, and bring to a boil, covered. Add carrots, do not stir.

Cover and simmer over low–medium heat for 30 minutes or until carrots are tender. Add prepared quinoa to stew, stir in salt and water as needed to achieve desired taste and consistency. Raise heat until stew is briskly bubbling. Fill the bottom half of large soup bowls with fresh spinach leaves. Spoon stew over spinach and serve.

Scallion Brown Rice

This recipe is from the highly acclaimed DASH Diet developed by the National Heart, Lung and Blood Institute, a department of the National Institutes of Health.

SERVES 5.

Ingredients
4 ½ cups cooked brown rice (cooked in unsalted water)
1 ½ teaspoons bouillon granules, low-sodium
¼ cup scallions (green onions), chopped

Procedure
Cook rice according to directions on the package. Combine the cooked rice, bouillon granules, and scallions and mix well.

Measure 1-cup portions and serve.

Meet the World's Healthiest Diet

Thre must be a million diets out there.

But we Americans keep getting fatter and sicker all the time. It is a full-blown red alert, "hair on fire" national emergency.

So I asked some of America's greatest, most distinguished health and nutrition experts a simple question: What are the best diets?

You'd be amazed by what they *didn't* say.

They didn't recommend any of the popular diet plans you see advertised on TV, with the exception of Weight Watchers, which gets good marks for its emphasis on calorie awareness and healthy eating.

They didn't recommend any of the fad diet books touting things like low carbs, high protein, meal timing, secret ingredients, flavor combining, coconuts, maple syrup and cayenne pepper drinks, diet bars, pills, or shakes. They didn't recommend fasting, cleansing, detoxing, colonics, or diets that cut out food groups.

Based on the research they've reviewed and the science they know, these experts really don't like the idea of diets much at all, when "diet" is defined as a restrictive program with lots of rules.

But the experts did identify several dietary patterns that they really like, which led me to a terrible realization about diets—*the diets most admired by experts are often the diets you rarely hear of, and never see advertised on TV.*

Two dietary approaches popped up repeatedly in the experts' comments and studies as models of healthy eating that, when combined with regular physical activity, can help you fight disease, achieve a healthy body weight, and Live Well (see the resources section at the back of this book for links to more information): The U.S. Dietary Guidelines for Americans issued in 2005, and the DASH diet (Dietary Approaches to Stop Hypertension) from the National Institutes of Health.

And when you ask the greatest medical and scientific experts to pick a single dietary approach that comes close to a gold standard of healthy nutrition, many of them agree on the Mediterranean diet. It may be the healthiest dietary pattern on Earth. In 2006, a team of scientists wrote in the journal *Nutrition Reviews* that "there is now evidence that the Mediterranean diet benefits not only the risk for coronary heart disease but also cancer occurrence, total mortality, and longevity."

The "Mediterranean diet" refers not to a diet book or a diet product, or even to a single strict diet, but to the traditional healthy eating *patterns* of Mediterranean countries like Greece, southern Italy, Crete, and Spain. (Unfortunately, heart disease and obesity are on the rise among many Mediterranean people, who are eating more calories, refined carbohydrates, and saturated fats—and getting less exercise. In other words, they're veering away from the Mediterranean diet!)

A typical traditional healthy Mediterranean diet pattern looks like this:

- high consumption of fruits, vegetables, bread and other cereals (often unrefined), potatoes, beans, nuts, and seeds
- foods like olive oil and fish as the major sources of good mono-unsaturated fat
- more fish eaten than red meat

- dairy products (usually cheese or yogurt) and poultry enjoyed in low-to-moderate amounts
- wine enjoyed in low-to-moderate amounts, generally with meals
- eggs eaten zero to four times a week

Since the 1960s, research has indicated that despite a fairly high fat intake (as much as 35 percent of calories), key Mediterranean countries enjoyed very low rates of coronary heart disease and high life expectancy. Ever since then, scientists have been trying to figure out the secret.

It's a great medical detective story, but scientists haven't cracked the case yet—they haven't really figured out precisely why the Mediterranean diet confers health benefits. At first, they thought the key was that the diet is relatively low in saturated fat, at under 8 percent of total calories. Recently, attention has shifted toward the possible protective effects of low-to-moderate wine consumption enjoyed in Mediterranean countries (usually with meals). But many experts are now most excited about two ideas:

- The benefits of the Mediterranean diet may come from the overall patterns of the diet working in a synergistic symphony, perhaps enhanced by lifestyle factors like strong family and community ties, and more physical activity.
- One of the most healthful benefits of the Mediterranean diet may be olive oil, which contains good monounsaturated fat, may reduce oxidative stress, and may protect against cardiovascular disease, several types of cancer, and age-related cognitive decline associated with Alzheimer's disease.

This Mediterranean diet chart is not a strict diet to follow, but an example of an ultrahealthy lifestyle pattern that helps many Mediterranean people enjoy good health and high longevity.

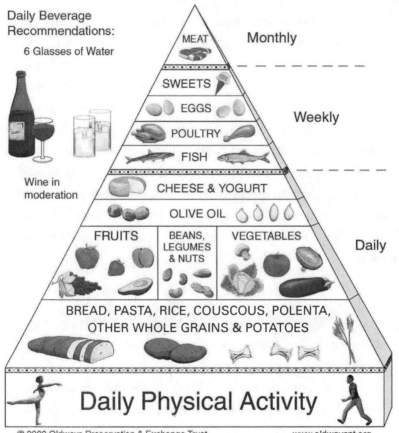

THE TRADITIONAL MEDITERRANEAN HEALTHY DIET PYRAMID

Daily Beverage Recommendations:

6 Glasses of Water

Wine in moderation

MEAT — Monthly

SWEETS

EGGS

POULTRY

FISH — Weekly

CHEESE & YOGURT

OLIVE OIL

FRUITS | BEANS, LEGUMES & NUTS | VEGETABLES — Daily

BREAD, PASTA, RICE, COUSCOUS, POLENTA, OTHER WHOLE GRAINS & POTATOES

Daily Physical Activity

The American Heart Association advises that if you do drink, you limit your daily intake to one drink for a woman, two for a man. In his book *Eat, Drink, and Be Healthy,* Dr. Walter Willett of the Harvard School of Public Health wrote that evidence suggests that one drink a day for women and one or two for men cuts the chances of having a heart attack or dying from heart disease by about a third, as well as reducing the risk of a clot-caused (ischemic) stroke. He added that a little alcohol can be beneficial, but "a lot can destroy the liver, lead to various cancers,* boost blood pressure, trigger bleeding (hemorrhagic) strokes, progressively weaken the heart muscle, scramble the brain, harm unborn children, and damage lives." He concluded, "If you don't drink alcohol, you shouldn't feel compelled to start," and "if you already drink alcohol, keep it moderate."

LIVING WELL CHECKOFF: DAY 7

I'm going to start applying some of the healthy lessons of the Mediterranean diet in my life—like eating plenty of produce and whole grains, and using extra-virgin olive oil.

Check Here: _____

---

*According to the American Cancer Society, alcohol is an established cause of cancers of the mouth, pharynx (throat), larynx (voice box), esophagus, liver, and breast, and may also increase the risk of colon and rectum cancer.

LIVING WELL MEDITERRANEAN-INSPIRED RECIPES

Steamed Artichoke with Spicy Extra-Virgin Olive Oil

Do not fear the artichoke! This vegetable is one of the most widely available, yet it's highly overlooked in the marketplace.

There are few joys in life as delightful as digging into a soft, steamy, creamy version of this supposedly intimidating vegetable.

Look for artichokes that have a deep green color and are heavy for their size. The leaves should be crisp and kind of squeak when you rub them together. Avoid dry-looking artichokes with split leaves or a lot of dark spots. A little discoloration on the edges of the leaves is okay. Wash just before cooking.

SERVES 2–4.

Ingredients

2 globe artichokes

1 lemon

1 clove garlic, thinly sliced

splash of white wine

pinch of finely ground black pepper

¼ cup extra-virgin olive oil

¼ teaspoon salt

¼ teaspoon red pepper flakes

Procedure

Cut off the bottom stems of the artichokes and rub the artichoke bottoms with the lemon. Cut about 2 inches off the top of the artichoke, and drizzle lemon juice over the top.

Using scissors, snip off the pointy ends of each outer leaf. This will keep you from getting stung later when the artichoke is ready to eat.

Using a stock pot big enough to fit and cover two artichokes, bring 3 inches of water to a boil. Add the garlic, wine, and pepper. Using tongs, carefully place artichokes top down into the pot. Simmer over low heat for 30–45 minutes. Pierce the bottom of the artichoke with a fork to check for doneness. If it is tender, the artichoke is cooked. Another indicator of a fully cooked artichoke is leaves that pull off easily. Using tongs, remove artichokes from the pot and set upright on a serving plate.

In a dipping bowl, whisk together olive oil, salt, and red pepper flakes.

To eat the artichoke, pull the leaves and dip the bottom tender part into the dipping oil and, using your teeth, pull off the tender "meat" from the bottom part of the leaves. Don't eat the rough tops. As more leaves come off, those toward the inside are more tender and the whole leaf can be eaten. Toward the heart of the artichoke, you will see fuzz. This should be scraped off with a spoon. What remains is the best part of all, the center or "heart" of the artichoke.

Raw Food Feast: Green Squash "Lasagna" with Basil Pesto, Sun-dried Tomato Sauce, and Cashew Cheese

I was really skeptical when I first heard of the idea of "raw foods pasta-style dishes" made not with pasta noodles and meat but with all veggies. Then I tried this recipe, and I was blown away by the complex feelings of satisfaction it delivered. This kind of dish is a staple in every raw-foods chef's repertoire. The easiest way to "hook" someone on trying some raw foods in their diet is to sit them down for an enjoyable feast of raw lasagna. Then tell them how fun it is to make.

SERVES 6.

CASHEW CHEESE

Ingredients

    2 cups raw cashews, soaked at least 2 hours
    2 tablespoons fresh lemon juice
    ½ clove raw garlic, chopped
    1 tablespoon raw onion
    ¼ teaspoon salt
    ½ cup water

Procedure

Rinse and strain cashews. Place the cashews, lemon juice, garlic, onion, and salt in a food processor and pulse until combined. Switch the food processor on, and very slowly add the water until the texture becomes smooth and creamy. Some water may remain unused. Transfer cashew cheese into a bowl, cover, and set aside in the refrigerator.

SUN-DRIED TOMATO SAUCE

Ingredients

> 2 cups sun-dried tomatoes, soaked at least 2 hours
> 10 grape tomatoes
> ⅛ sweet onion
> ½ clove raw garlic
> 1 tablespoon lemon juice
> 1 teaspoon low-sodium soy sauce
> 1–2 tablespoons agave nectar
> 2–4 tablespoons extra-virgin olive oil

Procedure

Squeeze sun-dried tomatoes dry. Add sun-dried tomatoes, grape tomatoes, onion, garlic, lemon juice, soy sauce, and agave to Vita-Mix and blend on low, gradually increasing to high speed. Slowly stream olive oil through hole in lid until tomato sauce reaches a smooth, spreadable consistency. Transfer tomato sauce into a bowl, cover, and set aside in the refrigerator.

BASIL PESTO

Ingredients

> 2 cups fresh basil leaves, packed
> ⅓ cup raw walnuts
> ½ cup extra-virgin olive oil
> 3 medium-sized garlic cloves, minced
> Salt and freshly ground black pepper to taste

Procedure

Pulse ingredients in a food processor until a desired chunky, spreadable consistency is achieved. Transfer pesto into a bowl, cover, and set aside in the refrigerator.

GREEN SQUASH LASAGNA

Ingredients

    4 large, wide, green squash (zucchini), ends removed

    Sun-dried Tomato Sauce

    Cashew Cheese

    Basil Pesto

    3 tablespoons extra-virgin olive oil

    ¼ teaspoon salt

    1 tablespoon fresh marjoram, finely chopped

    1 tablespoon fresh parsley, finely chopped

    1 tablespoon fresh thyme, stemmed

    6 large tomatoes, sliced into ¼-inch rounds

    6 fresh basil leaves

    freshly ground black pepper

Procedure

Using a mandoline or vegetable peeler, cut the squash lengthwise into lasagna noodle–like strips and begin to line the bottom of a 9-X-13-inch baking dish with a single layer of squash slices. It helps to slightly overlap slices. In 6 equally centered sections, spoon a dollop of each: Tomato Sauce, Cashew Cheese, and Pesto, side by side. Spoon a light coating of olive oil on top. Then sprinkle on a pinch of salt and a dusting of fresh herbs. Cover each section with a slice of tomato and press gently. Add another layer of squash over the length of the baking dish and repeat the addition of cheese, sauce, pesto, oil, salt, herbs, and then tomatoes. Repeat layering once more until 6 bare tomato slices are exposed. Garnish each tomato slice with sauce, cheese, and pesto side by side in the fashion of the Italian flag. Using a chef's knife, slice lasagna into 6 sections and spoon onto plates using a spatula. Garnish with a tuft of freshly sliced strips of basil and dust with black pepper.

Olive Energy Salad

Here's an action-packed salad that Chef Mike has whipped up for me between tapings of my show, when I need extra energy. When I'm finished chowing down on my first serving, I usually have one thing to say: "Give me more!"

SERVES 4–6.

Ingredients

1 cup pitted olives, any style

2 pounds vine-ripened tomatoes, cubed

1 small onion, diced

1 clove garlic, minced

1 tablespoon fresh lemon juice

1 tablespoon agave nectar or raw honey

1 head of basil, coarsely chopped

salt and pepper to taste

1 tablespoon toasted sesame seeds

Procedure

In a large mixing bowl, toss together olives, tomatoes, onion, garlic, lemon juice, sweetener, basil, salt, and pepper. Chill in the refrigerator for 30 minutes. Spoon into bowls. Then garnish with toasted sesame seeds. Enjoy.

LIVING WELL EXPERT
James Dillard, M.D.

Dr. James Dillard is the medical director of the Rosenthal Center for Complementary and Alternative Medicine at Columbia University and assistant clinical professor at Columbia University College of Physicians and Surgeons. He is also on the medical staff at the New York–Presbyterian Hospital, and attending physician at Beth Israel Medical Center in the Department of Pain Medicine and Palliative Care.

Dr. Dillard is the author of *The Chronic Pain Solution* and lectures on how to integrate complementary and alternative approaches into conventional medical delivery systems.

What makes Dr. Dillard very special is his unique background. He is one of the very few American doctors who have been trained in all three of these professions: medicine, acupuncture, and chiropractic. This proves to me that his mind is wide-open to conventional medicine as well as alternative therapies.

Dr. Dillard praises the benefits of a Mediterranean-style diet based on whole foods, which to me is the essence of the Living Well Code.

Dr. Dillard believes that for the 65 million Americans who suffer with chronic pain conditions, what you eat can make a big difference. In his book he writes about a version of the Mediterranean diet that he calls "the Anti-Inflammatory Diet," which he believes can really quiet down your nerves if you have chronic pain.

If you're eating a significant amount of processed foods, you're just not going to be healthy. You should eat a "whole-foods diet" that does not have processed foods in it.

In our culture we've gotten farther and farther away from the farm, from the patch where the food is grown.

Our food is increasingly processed and shipped around the country as much as two thousand miles. The more you separate yourself from food that is fresh and has just come out of the ground, the more you're going to lose nutrition, quality, and taste.

If you're living in an urban area, you can go to a farmers' market. If you're in a more rural area, try to get to know farmers near you who are actually growing your foods, so you know where your food is coming from.

Many health experts are advocating a diet that is close to the ground that is based upon whole foods, the kind of foods that people used to eat in the old days. Back then, you pulled a turnip out of the ground, you cooked it, and you ate it. That's a whole food.

Whole foods can have significant effects on your health. They tend to be healthy for us, and protect us from various kinds of illnesses, not just cancer, but also heart disease and degenerative illnesses.

Eating nothing but raw, uncooked foods is a plan that a certain number of people follow, and there have been books written about it. The problem is that there isn't any real compelling science to dictate that we should eat nothing but raw food. And besides, many important nutrients are released by gentle cooking.

As a matter of fact, there are some good examples of food that is actually much more nutritionally healthy when cooked. For example, fresh tomatoes have a component called lycopene that's gotten a lot of good press lately. If you eat a raw tomato, you don't absorb as much lycopene as you do if you cooked that tomato.

(continued)

Most of us are recommending the Mediterranean diet, which is based primarily around fresh vegetables, fresh fruits, and some whole grains, and a minimum of protein. Studies have indicated that people who eat the Mediterranean diet have much lower rates of cancer and heart disease. ■

LIVING WELL EXPERT
Ralph Sacco, M.D.

Dr. Ralph Sacco is professor and chairman of the department of neurology at the University of Miami, and previously served as director, Stroke and Critical Care Division at Columbia University Medical Center.

He is a leading authority on vascular diseases and the prevention of strokes, and serves on the board of directors of the American Heart Association and the American Academy of Neurology.

Vascular diseases are a massive threat to our health, affecting tens of millions of Americans. Here, Dr. Sacco tells us how to take charge and fight vascular diseases with diet and exercise.

Vascular disease is a big group of chronic diseases, including cardiovascular disease and stroke, that are affected by many diet and lifestyle factors.

Most studies have shown that Mediterranean diets, and diets rich in vegetables, fruits, and whole grains, are protective when it comes to the risk of vascular diseases.

Studies have also shown that diets high in sodium are deleterious because they can increase the risk of high blood pressure, which can contribute to heart disease and stroke.

We used to think of Alzheimer's disease as a neurodegenerative disease under genetic control. But the data is suggesting more and more that vascular risk factors are related to Alzheimer's disease.

High blood pressure, diabetes, and other vascular risk factors will also contribute to poor cognition from Alzheimer's and what we call vascular cognitive impairment, which is another big cause of losing memory with age.

Beyond diet, there are three lifestyle factors that affect vascular disease: exercise, smoking, and alcohol.

Being physically active is critical to reducing the risk of chronic vascular disease. Multiple studies have shown that starting physical activity at younger ages and hopefully continuing good patterns of physical activity as one ages are critical to reduce vascular risk.

There is some disagreement over exactly how much and what kinds of exercise are best. You don't have to be a marathon runner, but at least twenty to thirty minutes of exercise every day is a good target.

Smoking: just don't do it, ever. It's so clear that smoking is associated with multiple chronic diseases, like cancer and heart disease.

The third factor in lifestyle is alcohol.

I preach alcohol in moderation. Among other problems, excess alcohol will definitely increase the risk of stroke, it may increase heart disease, it affects the liver, it affects the nervous system in other ways, it can cause degeneration of parts of the brain and balance difficulty, and it can cause degeneration even in nerves and parts of the spinal cord. Moderate alcohol—often described as up to two drinks per day for men and one for women—may actually provide some beneficial vascular effects.

Some people are really into megavitamins, but it's hard to find studies that have shown definite benefits. ■

Energize Your Body

Small Steps:

- Be mindful of your calories in and calories out to work toward a healthy body weight.
- Gradually begin working toward the target of at least thirty to sixty minutes of moderate physical activity on most days of the week.

WEEK 2
ENERGIZE YOUR BODY

Small Steps:
- Be mindful of your "calories in" and "calories out," to work toward a healthy body weight.

- Start gradually working toward the target of thirty to sixty minutes of physical activity on most days of the week.

	MON	TUE	WED	THU	FRI	SAT	SUN
BREAKFAST							
LUNCH							
DINNER							
ALL OTHER: *Snacks, Lattes, Candy, Liquid Candy (Sugared Beverages), Office Munchies, etc.*							
PHYSICAL ACTIVITY TYPE:							
HOW MANY MINUTES:							

MY SPECIFIC PLANS TO LIVE WELL THIS WEEK:

The kinds of foods I'll enjoy:

The physical activities I'll enjoy:

The behaviors I'll make better:

The attitudes I'll make better:

Ways I'll help my family live well:

Learn the Living Well Calorie Formula

Let's get moving!

A healthy body weight is crucial to Living Well. And the key to achieving a Living Well body weight is quite simple, and unglamorous: you've got to balance the calories you consume with the calories you burn off. Calories are king.

So to truly Live Well physically, you've got to do two things—you've got to eat healthy, and you've got to energize your body on most days of the week, with at least thirty minutes of physical activity—and preferably sixty minutes—per day.

Week 1 of this 21-Day Living Well Program was about eating well. This week, Week 2, let's focus on energizing our body through physical activity and exercise.

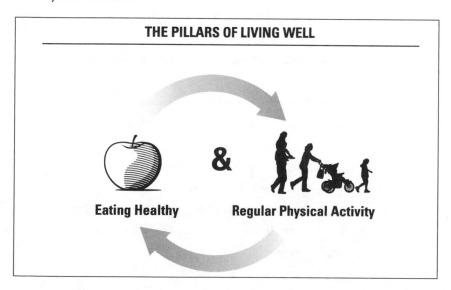

THE PILLARS OF LIVING WELL

Eating Healthy   &   Regular Physical Activity

I'm a physical, active person, and I thrive on that activity. You will, too. Physical activity supercharges your body by multiplying the impact of healthy eating in a self-supporting, positive loop.

I've been working out almost nonstop for over thirty years. I've worked with and interviewed hundreds of the best trainers, physical therapists, and exercise researchers in the world. A few years ago I wrote a bestselling book called *BodyChange* with the trainer Wini Linguvic. And I've learned twelve important things about exercise and physical activity:

Montel's 12 Lessons on Physical Activity

1. Exercise works. It can change your body and it can change your life.
2. You have control over how you look and how you feel.
3. The power you gain from exercise will support you in all aspects of your life.
4. Exercise is your gift to yourself, a time you should and will look forward to.
5. When you understand how good exercise makes you feel, it gets easier and more fun.
6. Exercise also gets easier as your body adapts. Soon you'll find that physical activity will become a way of life for you—one of the most enjoyable parts of your day.
7. Exercise is something you deserve that will enrich your life for years to come.
8. Progress doesn't happen overnight. Be patient and break your physical activity goals into small, manageable pieces. Keep track of your progress, celebrate your victories.
9. Keeping a fitness diary to chart your progress is a great idea—it will show you how far you have come.
10. Even a strong start can fizzle out after a few weeks. Motivation is the one thing that will keep you going through busy days, bad weather, and tired spells.

11. Get psyched! Your body loves and craves activity. Soon, you'll feel more energy, more strength, and less stress.

12. Shaking off excess weight takes time, but when you combine physical activity with a healthy eating plan—it can absolutely happen!

Some fad diets do work for a little while, but only because they put a cork on your daily calorie intake, not from any magic combination of foods. The basic physical formula for your weight control is amazingly simple: balance your calories in from food and drink with your calories out from physical activity.

That is the magic, irrevocable equation for managing your weight. "It's not low fat vs. low carb," wrote Dr. Dean Ornish, director of the Preventive Medicine Research Institute. "You can eat fewer calories by eating less food—which is why you can lose weight on any diet that restricts entire categories of foods or limits portion sizes—but you may get hungry and gain it back." As Dr. Walter Willett and the cookbook author Mollie Katzen put it in their book *Eat, Drink, and Weigh Less*: "If you're trying to lose weight, don't just indiscriminately cut out fat, carbohydrates or protein. Eat the right kinds of each, and burn more calories than you eat."

"Weight loss is 100 percent contingent upon achieving a calorie deficit," according to the Mount Sinai Medical Center senior clinical dietitian Rebecca Blake, who told the January 2, 2007, *New York Daily News* that, for example, "If the Atkins diet does work for an individual, it is entirely because they have achieved a calorie deficit," not because of a manipulation of carbs in the diet. "The laws of physics govern weight loss and weight gain," agrees the nutritionist Carla Wolper at St. Luke's New York Obesity Research Center. "And physics looks at energy, which is equal to calories. Physics has not heard of the Atkins diet."

It's as basic as balancing your checkbook. Here's how the formula works:

The Living Well Formula
for Weight Loss and Weight Control

Balance Your Calories In/Calories Out, or Energy In/Energy Out

Calories Consumed > Calories Burned off = Weight Gain

Calories Consumed < Calories Burned off = Weight Loss

Calories Consumed = Calories Burned off = Weight Control

THE LIVING WELL FORMULA

GAINING WEIGHT

Calories In > Calories Out

You will gain weight when the calories you eat and drink are greater than the calories you burn.

LOSING WEIGHT

Calories In < Calories Out

You will lose weight when the calories you eat and drink are less than the calories you burn.

MAINTAINING WEIGHT

Calories In = Calories Out

Your weight will stay the same when the calories you eat and drink equal the calories you burn.

You can boil the Living Well formula down to four words: *eat better, move more.* You've got to combine healthy eating with physical activity. And physical activity includes these options, which can add up to the target of thirty to sixty minutes per day on most days of the week:

- concentrated, structured exercises, like brisk walking or exercises you do in a gym
- "exercise snacks" of short bursts of activity of at least ten minutes, like shorter power walks, climbing stairs, gardening, and vacuuming

It's important for you to know that experts see the Living Well benefits of healthy eating and physical activity as linked and interdependent: you can't do just one or the other if you want the best results. Healthy eating helps you lose weight and physical activity helps you keep it off. Sticking with the two together over the long term is what helps you truly Live Well for life.

Montel's Tips for Calorie Awareness

Starting today, start making "calorie awareness" a part of your daily routine:

- You don't have to obsess or feel guilty over every single calorie—just make a point of being aware of the scale of calories you consume every day.
- Check nutrition labels and keep a rough running total of your calories in through the course of your day.
- If you're feeling really bold, at restaurants and takeouts, ask for calorie information. If they won't give it to you, tell them you'll go somewhere else until they do.
- Jot down all your food, beverages, and snacks in the Living Well Action Plan.
- Also jot down your physical activities in the Living Well Action Plan.
- To see specifically how many calories per day you need based on your height, weight, and activity level, go to the Web site www.mypyramid.gov and click on MyPyramid Plan.

LIVING WELL CHECKOFF: DAY 8

I will work to achieve and maintain a healthy body weight over time by being calorie aware, and balancing my calories in through food and beverages with my calories out through physical activity.

Check Here: _____

What the Experts Say

A combination of regular exercise and a mostly plant-based diet is the key to maintaining a healthy body weight.

—AMERICAN INSTITUTE FOR CANCER RESEARCH

Maintaining a healthy weight isn't about going on a diet and coming off a diet when you reach your target weight. It is about adopting skills that change your eating habits for life.

—DR. BECKIE LANG, ASSOCIATION FOR THE
STUDY OF OBESITY, UK

From the Dietary Guidelines for Americans, 2005:
• Calorie intake and physical activity go hand in hand in controlling weight. Most Americans need to reduce the amount of calories they consume.
• When it comes to weight control, calories count—not the proportions of carbohydrate, fat, and protein in the diet.
• Calories expended must equal calories consumed to stay at the same weight. A deficit can be achieved by eating less, being more active physically, or combining the two.
• Since many adults gain weight slowly over time, even a small calorie deficit can help you avoid weight gain. For example, a calorie deficit of 50 to 100 calories per day would enable many adults to maintain their weight rather than continuing to gain weight each year.

• Small changes maintained over time can make a big difference in body weight.

• Monitoring weight regularly helps you know if you need to adjust your food intake or amount of physical activity to maintain your weight.

• Limiting portion sizes often helps reduce calorie intake, especially if the food is high in calorie density.

• On the other hand, consuming large portions of raw vegetables or low-fat soups may help limit your intake of other foods that are more calorie-dense.

• The healthiest way to reduce calorie intake is to reduce your intake of added sugars, solid fats, and alcohol—they all provide calories, but they do not provide essential nutrients.

• The recommended ranges for fat calories (20 to 35 percent of total calories), carbohydrate calories (45 to 65 percent of total calories), and protein calories (10 to 35 percent of total calories) provide sufficient flexibility to accommodate weight maintenance for a wide variety of body sizes and food preferences.

LIVING WELL EXPERT
James O. Hill, Ph.D.

Dr. James O. Hill is professor of pediatrics and medicine and director of the Center for Human Nutrition at the University of Colorado at Denver Health Sciences Center.

We've all heard by now that diets don't work, and that people often put more weight back on after they've stopped dieting. It seems to be a pretty bleak, disappointing picture.

(continued)

But Dr. Hill is here with terrific news: many people actually do successfully lose major weight, and keep it off for the long haul. He has the research, and the tips, to prove it. Dr. Hill is the cofounder of the National Weight Control Registry, a remarkable database of over five thousand people who have lost thirty pounds or more and kept it off for over a year.

Dr. Hill is one of the country's leading experts on successful weight loss, obesity, and the health benefits of physical activity. He is the cofounder of America on the Move, a national initiative that aims to inspire Americans to make small changes in how much they eat and how much they move to prevent weight gain. He is also the author of *The Step Diet Book*.

What's fascinating about Dr. Hill is how much emphasis he places on exercise as a totally crucial strategy for your health. It's practically a magic drug! Dr. Hill is absolutely right—I'm fifty-one years old, and I'm training harder now than when I was in my twenties. And I feel the benefits every single day.

If physical activity came in a pill it would truly be a miracle drug. When it comes to exercise, anything you do is good.

One of the biggest things we've learned from the National Weight Control Registry is that losing weight is different from keeping it off. The public still doesn't get this.

We can succeed pretty easily with taking the weight off, but weight-loss maintenance is harder.

There are lots of ways to lose weight that are OK as long as you realize weight loss is a temporary step. But then you have to find a way to live your life forever—and that's where people fail way more than they succeed.

The key is physical activity. At the end of the day, what we're talking about are balances. Everywhere throughout the world of health, nutrition, and wellness, you're going to come to this concept of balance.

About two-thirds of Americans get little or no physical activity. I believe that if you're that sedentary, there's no way you're going to be healthy. You can't be healthy with diet alone.

The first thing you have to do is increase activity. What activity does is get you into the range where it is feasible for you to achieve balance with diet.

Walking and other physical activities do many things. First of all, they help with energy balance: balancing your calories in with calories out.

If you're at a very low level of activity, the only way you can balance your energy in with energy out is through food restriction. But you can't do that for very long. Human beings are not set up to food-restrict. So unless you increase your activity, you aren't going to be able to balance energy. Increasing activity allows you to eat an amount of food you can be satisfied with over the long term.

Second, physical activity has independent effects over and above weight management.

Exercise improves glucose metabolism, it helps prevent diabetes, and it improves heart health. You get a double bang for your buck: better weight management, and also better direct management of the risk factors for chronic disease.

And then finally, it has positive effects on mood, fighting depression and making you feel better.

This is all based on solid evidence, a wealth of data. If we could get people to get physically active, we know what's going to happen—they're going to lower their weight and reduce their risk for health problems.

(continued)

Start where you are now, and work up gradually. Most people don't even get ten minutes of physical activity a day, so if you expect all of a sudden to get ninety minutes, you're going to fail. Increase your amount of daily steps gradually. Do it throughout the day. If you get to a meeting five minutes early, take a walk.

If you don't have sidewalks in your neighborhood, is there a park or a ball field nearby? Or even a Wal-Mart you can walk around?

It really is worth it. The impact of physical activity is so positive, but you've got to be in this for the long run.

After you're walking consistently, adding something like weight lifting is great. It helps in weight management; it helps in being able to maintain functionality as you age. But I wouldn't start out there because I think it's hard for many people to go from doing nothing to lifting weights.

We've learned good news and bad news at the National Weight Loss Registry.

The bad news is it really does require changing your life.

The good news is that people can do it.

There's no similarity in how the successful losers lost the weight. They're not keeping the weight off with popular diet plans like Atkins, Zone, and South Beach. Some may have lost weight on those diets, but they're not using those diets over the long term to keep weight off.

Among people in the Registry who have lost weight and kept it off, the most critical thing is their level of physical activity. More than 90 percent of these people have high levels of physical activity: an average of sixty to ninety minutes a day. That speaks pretty powerfully to me.

You should know that it takes a lot less physical activity to keep from gaining weight in the first place than it does to keep the weight off once you've gained it. You pay a penalty for being obese. For most people an extra fifteen minutes a day of activity will prevent weight gain, but once you get obese and then lose weight, you need sixty to ninety minutes to maintain.

There's a lot of research out there showing that physical activity combined with a low-fat diet is a logical strategy to keep weight off. You get multiple benefits from healthy eating. You get low calorie density from fruit, vegetables, and whole grains, which means you'll overeat less. Plus, the good stuff in fruits and vegetables tends to promote health, and helps you avoid the chronic diseases like diabetes and heart disease, independently of weight. So with diet and exercise you get a double bang for your buck.

Healthy eating allows people to maintain a healthy weight and prevent diabetes and heart disease, and it's the kind of diet we ought to be recommending to everybody.

This is an important point: let's not just single out the obese people and say, "You guys need to eat healthy and get physically active."

This is for everybody. ■

Feel the Joy of Regular Physical Activity

I've had mountain highs, and I've had rock bottoms.

Mountain highs are those golden days when the stars are aligned, the skies are deep blue, God is on your shoulder, and something magnificent happens—you meet your future spouse, your son or daughter makes you proud, or someone tells you how much you mean to him.

Then you've got the rock-bottom days, hopefully not too many of them, when you hit a bump, fly off the track, and crash into a brick wall.

Without a doubt, the worst rock-bottom day in my life was the day I was diagnosed with multiple sclerosis.

Back in the early 1990s, I was on a roll. I was working out every day. My career was beginning to take off. But every couple of years, I experienced this really crazy excruciating pain in my legs and in my feet. It was bad enough, and lasted long enough, that I went to various doctors and had it checked out.

One doctor after another said the exact same thing: "You're working out too much." Their conclusion was always the same: "Just take it easy for a while. It'll pass." Well, you know what? I would. I'd ease up on my workouts, and for a few months the pain would go away. Problem solved, right? No. It kept coming back.

Finally, in 1999, I saw a specialist. He checked me out. Without any warning he said, "I'm sorry I've got to tell you this, but you've got MS.

Life's going to change for you. You're not going to be able to do your show, because I think it's maybe too stressful. You're going to have to avoid all stressful office situations. You need to stop working out, too, because it's just putting too much of a load on your nervous system. It's gonna destroy you." The message I got from this doctor was "It's all over. You're a dead man."

For a while I was too stunned to cry. It felt like a bad science fiction movie where someone's body is suddenly possessed by an alien force. But it was real, it was happening to me, and it was my body that was condemned.

I could have curled up in a ball right then and there and I could have died. But I didn't. *How dare you define me?* I thought. *Am I going to walk out of this office a different person from when I walked in, just because of some words that you've said?*

Go home and die? I decided to go home and live instead. Every single day, I tell myself I'm going to be the person who owns the definition of who I am, nobody else.

So after some really dark days, I took charge, opened my mind to floodgates of new knowledge, research, and information gathering—and I hit the gym.

I work out like my life depends on it.

You are a physically active person, whether you realize it or not. I guarantee it! Like your caveman ancestors, you are genetically engineered to move your body, chase your spouse, run after your kids, jump, climb, forage, wander, power walk, and lift weights.

When you propel yourself into enjoying regular physical exercise, you are fulfilling your biological destiny. By the way, I use the terms "exercise" and "physical activity" fairly interchangeably. Exercise means a structured program, and physical activity also includes unstructured physical movements you accumulate through the day. Both of them give you great benefits when performed at moderate intensity or more, in periods of ten minutes or more.

Exercise alone usually won't help you lose a great deal of weight. In fact, healthy eating with calorie control is a more efficient way of melting excess pounds off. But sustained physical activity is crucial to maintaining a healthy weight and preventing weight regain. And like healthy eating, it also helps you fight the risks of many diseases.

And then there's that indescribable feeling of physical joy that exercise can often give you: it can make you feel totally spectacular. Nowadays, my mountain high days come fast and furious when I exercise.

No matter where you are in life, whether you're in perfect health or you have a medical challenge, I think regular physical activity is one of your magic bullets for Living Well. Don't think of it as an optional choice, or as a "something I'll have to find the time for someday" thing. Finding the motivation and time for it is essential—it's a must do!

In 2006 the U.S. Department of Health and Human Services issued some amazing statistics:

- Chronic diseases account for seven of every ten U.S. deaths and for more than 60 percent of medical care expenditures.
- Much of the chronic disease burden is preventable.
- Physical inactivity and unhealthy eating contribute to obesity, cancer, cardiovascular disease, and diabetes, which together are responsible for at least 300,000 deaths each year.
- Only tobacco use causes more preventable deaths in the United States.
- People who avoid the behaviors that increase their risk for chronic diseases can expect to live healthier and longer lives.
- Regular physical activity substantially reduces the risk of dying of coronary heart disease, the nation's leading cause of death, and decreases the risk of developing colon cancer, type 2 diabetes, and high blood pressure.
- Regular physical activity also helps to control weight; contributes to healthy bones, muscles, and joints; reduces falls among the elderly;

helps to relieve the pain of arthritis; reduces symptoms of anxiety and depression; and is associated with fewer hospitalizations, physician visits, and medications.

• Moreover, physical activity need not be strenuous to be beneficial; people of all ages benefit from moderate physical activity, such as thirty minutes of brisk walking on five or more days a week.

• Despite the proven benefits of physical activity, more than 60 percent of American adults do not get enough physical activity to provide health benefits.

• More than 25 percent are not active at all in their leisure time. Activity decreases with age and is less common among women than men and among those with lower income and less education.

• Insufficient physical activity is not limited to adults. More than a third of young people in grades 9–12 do not regularly engage in vigorous physical activity. Daily participation in high school physical education classes dropped from 42 percent in 1991 to 29 percent in 1999.

By the way, if you have kids, here's a shocker—the latest U.S. Dietary Guidelines for Americans declare:

Children and adolescents need at least sixty minutes of moderate-to-vigorous physical activity on most days for the maintenance of good health and fitness and for healthy weight gain during growth.

Wait a minute—stop the presses! Can you believe that? How many kids and teenagers do you know who are getting at least sixty minutes of exercise a day on most days? Are you kidding? Our schools are slashing physical education programs left and right, and we're in the midst of a raging national epidemic of childhood obesity! How are we supposed to do this?

Well, it's our responsibility. We have to make it happen. Repeat after me, loud and clear: "Our kids must get a minimum of at least sixty minutes of moderate-to-vigorous physical activity on most days of the week."

I want you and your kids to write that sentence in bold Magic Marker on a sheet of paper—and tape it to the refrigerator. It is their crucial new Living Well commandment to work toward.

We have to get over ourselves, stop bellyaching about how impossible things are, take charge, and as the great Nike ad campaign proclaimed, *just do it.*

If you've got the time to watch TV every day, then you can definitely find some time for your family to enjoy some physical activity!

Don't your kids deserve a healthy life?

15 Ways Your Life Can Be Transformed by Regular Physical Activity

The list of benefits you can enjoy when you get moving is absolutely incredible. According to the World Health Organization and other health authorities, regular physical activity:

1. Reduces the risk of dying prematurely and reduces the risk of dying from heart disease or stroke, which are responsible for one-third of all deaths.
2. Reduces the risk of developing heart disease or colon cancer by up to 50 percent.
3. May protect against breast and lung cancers.
4. Reduces the risk of developing type 2 diabetes 50 percent.
5. Helps to prevent/reduce hypertension.
6. Helps to prevent/reduce osteoporosis, reducing the risk of hip fracture by up to 50 percent in women.
7. Reduces the risk of developing lower back pain.
8. Promotes psychological well-being, reduces stress, anxiety, and feelings of depression and loneliness.
9. Protects against age-related memory loss.

10. Helps prevent or control risky behaviors, especially among children and young people, like tobacco, alcohol, or other substance use, unhealthy diet, or violence.
11. Helps control weight and lower the risk of becoming obese by 50 percent compared to people with sedentary lifestyles.
12. Helps build and maintain healthy bones, muscles, and joints and makes people with chronic, disabling conditions improve their stamina.
13. Can help in the management of painful conditions, like back pain or knee pain.
14. Improves flexibility, strength, balance, and endurance.
15. Through its link to weight control, physical activity may also help fight obesity-related cancers, such as those of the endometrium (lining of the uterus), kidney, breast (in postmenopausal women), colon, pancreas, and prostate, according to the American Institute of Cancer Research (AICR).

The great news is you don't have to train like an Olympic contender to enjoy the benefits of physical activity. At least thirty minutes of moderate physical activity on most days of the week is enough to bring many of these effects.

More than thirty minutes of moderate-to-vigorous physical activity on most days gives you extra health benefits. And many adults may need up to sixty or ninety minutes of moderate-to-vigorous physical activity on most days to prevent unhealthy weight gain. (Moderate-intensity exercise means you'll breathe harder and find it harder to talk, but you should still be able to carry on a conversation.)

To hit a target of sixty minutes a day of moderate physical activity is easier than you think. You can get started just by paying attention to ways of squeezing out more activity from your daily life. According to the American Institute for Cancer Research, you can, for example, break the time down into workable segments, or "exercise snacks," and before you know it, you've hit your daily goal. An exercise snack is a physical activity performed at moderate intensity for at least ten minutes.

Here's one example:

Exercise Snack	Minutes of Moderate Exercise
Take the dog for a brisk walk in the morning	10 minutes
Park the car at the edge of the lot and briskly walk to the store	10 minutes
Take the stairs at work instead of riding the elevator	10 minutes
Do some gardening or play softball with the kids after school	30 minutes
	Grand total: 60 minutes

In terms of more structured activities, vigorous physical activity delivers greater physical fitness benefits and burns more calories than moderate physical activity.

Vigorous Physical Activity	Calories Burned per Hour
Running/jogging	590
Bicycling (more than 10 mph)	590
Swimming (slow freestyle laps)	510
Aerobics	480
Walking (4.5 mph)	460
Heavy yard work (like chopping wood)	440
Weight lifting (vigorous workout)	440
Basketball (vigorous)	440

Moderate Physical Activity	Calories Burned per Hour
Hiking	370
Light gardening/yard work	330
Dancing	330
Golf (walking and carrying clubs)	330
Bicycling (less than 10 mph)	290
Walking (3.5 mph)	280
Weight lifting (light workout)	220
Stretching	180

Source: National Institutes of Health. These are the average number of calories a 154-pound person will burn, per hour, for each activity. A lighter person will burn fewer calories; a heavier person will burn more.

There are three major types of structured physical activity: *aerobic/ cardiovascular, resistance/strength, and flexibility.* They are all important parts of a physical fitness program, and they work together to reinforce each other. For instance, resistance exercises can help you obtain the muscle strength, balance, and coordination to perform your aerobic activities effectively.

Aerobic and cardiovascular activity benefits the heart most. It uses large muscle groups and causes your body to use more oxygen than it would normally. *Examples*: brisk walking, jogging, and bicycling.

Resistance and strength training strengthens muscles and bones, tones muscles, and improves your balance and coordination. They focus on major muscle groups like the legs, chest, and back. Experts suggest strength training on two or three days each week, with a full day of rest in between workouts to let your body recharge. *Examples:* weight training, using resistance bands, using stability or medicine balls, performing abdominal crunches and push-ups.

Flexibility exercises limber up your muscles and keep your joints flexible.

Putting it all together, here's a sample weekly schedule that combines all three categories:

Sample Activity Program: Weekly Schedule			
Sunday	aerobic		flexibility
Monday	aerobic	strength	flexibility
Tuesday	aerobic		flexibility
Wednesday	aerobic	strength	flexibility
Thursday	aerobic		flexibility
Friday	aerobic	strength	flexibility
Saturday		day off	

Source: Adapted from the National Institutes of Health.

Other terrific exercises that can lower stress, build strength, flexibility, and balance, increase energy, and deliver excellent fitness benefits include *yoga*, *Pilates*, and *tai chi*. I've tried them all and I urge you to check them out, see if you like them, and work them into your life.

Montel's Living Well Physical Activity Tips

• Get your doctor's opinion and OK before starting an exercise program.

• Start slowly and go for slow, steady progress. Gradually work toward the thirty- and sixty-minute goals over weeks and months. If you try too much too fast, you increase the risk of injury.

• If you feel any pain during exercise, stop right away and be sure to consult your doctor. Uncomfortable stiffness, dizziness, or severe breathlessness are also signs that you should stop and get medical attention.

• Stay hydrated: drink fluids, especially water, before, during, and after your exercise and physical activity.

- Consider hooking up with a certified personal trainer who can design a personalized approach for you. Look for a personal trainer with a degree in exercise physiology, or who is certified through a professional group like the American College of Sports Medicine, American Council on Exercise, or National Strength and Conditioning Association.
- *Before you exercise, "warm up" with about five minutes of walking, marching in place, or a less strenuous version of the activity you're about to do.* Note: this is not stretching. A warm-up and stretching (see below) are two different things.
- At the end of the exercise, slow down gradually with five minutes of a similar cooldown. For example, if you're finishing off a run, slow down to a jog, then a walk.
- Finally, if you want to stretch, *do your stretching at the end of your workout* while your muscles are warm and limber.

What the Experts Recommend

In 2007, the American College of Sports Medicine and the American Heart Association got together to recommend these tips for physical activity to promote and maintain health, and reduce risk of chronic disease and premature death:

- All healthy adults ages eighteen to sixty-five years need moderate-intensity aerobic physical activity for at least thirty minutes on five days each week or vigorous-intensity aerobic physical activity for at least twenty minutes on three days each week. Aerobic activity is needed in addition to routine activities of daily life.
- Moderate-intensity aerobic activity is described as generally equivalent to a brisk walk, or activity that noticeably accelerates the heart rate.
- Vigorous-intensity activity is exemplified by jogging, and causes rapid breathing and a substantial increase in heart rate.
- Moderate- or vigorous-intensity activities performed as a part of daily

life (for example, brisk walking to work, gardening with a shovel, carpentry) performed in bouts of ten minutes or more can be counted toward the recommendation.

• In addition, every adult should perform activities that maintain or increase muscular strength and endurance for at least two days each week. It is recommended that 8–10 exercises using the major muscle groups be performed on two nonconsecutive days. To maximize strength development, a resistance (weight) should be used for 8–12 repetitions of each exercise.

LIVING WELL CHECKOFFS: DAY 9

• Starting today, I will think of myself as a fit, active, powerful person. I can be and I will be!

Check Here: _____

• I believe that exercise should not be a chore. It is a pathway to beautiful health and physical joy.

Check Here: _____

• Beginning today, I will start working gradually toward the goal of thirty to sixty minutes of moderate-to-vigorous physical activity per day on most days of the week.

Check Here: _____

LIVING WELL EXPERT
Laurence S. Sperling, M.D.

Dr. Laurence S. Sperling is the founder and director of preventive cardiology at the Emory University Clinic, codirector of the cardiovascular disease fellowship program at Emory, and director of the Emory Heartwise Risk Reduction Program. He is an associate professor of medicine (cardiology) at the Emory University School of Medicine.

I asked Dr. Sperling to speak to us because he is a top authority on fighting America's number-one killer, cardiovascular disease, and because he was a lead author of a major review article, "Diets and Cardiovascular Disease: An Evidence-based Assessment," which appeared in the May 2005 issue of the *Journal of the American College of Cardiology.*

Diet, exercise, and lifestyle are very powerful tools for health, potentially more powerful in totality than any of the medical therapies we have.

The American diet right now is a disaster. It's killing people.

The scary thing is a lot of these dietary habits are spreading now to third-world countries and areas of the world that haven't seen them before, like China, Russia, and India. So we're looking toward a worldwide epidemic of problems like diabetes and heart disease.

For many people, the benefits of following a healthy dietary pattern like the Mediterranean diet or the DASH diet (Dietary Approaches to Stop Hypertension) will be cardiovascular health, cancer protection, improvement of blood pressure, reducing risk for diabetes, hopefully weight reduction and having protection from a lot of chronic disease processes, and even helping in the treatment of a lot of chronic disease processes.

Unfortunately, behavioral and lifestyle changes are not easy for human beings. It's hard for somebody to overhaul what they have

(continued)

done for the last fifty years overnight. But you can begin to change gradually. You have to break things up into manageable concepts and manageable goals.

You can lose weight in the short term on any type of gimmicky quick-fix fad diet. But most of the time you'll gain that weight right back. So instead of a short-term approach where you lose twenty pounds in a month, you should look for permanent changes and really sustainable behavioral changes.

Focus on simple things like portion size, and balancing your calories in with your calories out.

Exercise is a very potent therapy for all kinds of disease processes. It is a very healthy preventive therapy and it's probably one of the most potent antioxidants we know of. It ameliorates the process called oxidative stress, and oxidative stresses are tied to lots of disease processes, like heart disease, diabetes, and rheumatologic disorders. I also believe it is tied to some degree to multiple sclerosis and the aging process in general.

Exercise is ten thousand times more potent an antioxidant than vitamin C and vitamin E. Ten years ago, all the cardiologists were telling their patients to take vitamin C and vitamin E. But then, well-designed clinical research studies showed there's no benefit from vitamin E and C supplements.

Patients come into my office with a bag of health-food supplements and ask, "Dr. Sperling, what do you think of these?" A lot of these supplements have no legitimate scientific studies to warrant somebody taking them. I tell patients, "Instead of taking a bag of pills, you should eat well, and exercise regularly." ■

Get Up, Get Out, and Power Walk

Stop reading this book.

Right now, I want you to stop reading this book, go put your sneakers on, get outside and take a thirty-minute walk, then come back. Warm up by walking at a normal pace for five minutes, then walk briskly for twenty minutes, then cool down by walking at a normal pace for the final five minutes. "Brisk" means walking fast, faster than a recreational stroll and slower than a race walk, or about three to four miles an hour.

I mean it. Put the book down, lace up, and get moving, OK?

I'll see you when you get back.

There—didn't that feel great?

You just performed a power walk, one of the easiest, safest, and most enjoyable aerobic exercises in the world. Brisk walking is an example of moderate physical activity, so it counts toward the Living Well Code target of thirty to sixty minutes a day of moderate-intensity physical activity on most days of the week. It gives you terrific health benefits. And if you're not getting regular exercise, power walking is a great way to start.

"Walking may be as close to a magic bullet as you'll find in modern medicine," Dr. JoAnn Manson, a professor of medicine at Harvard Medical School, told the *Los Angeles Times* last year. "If there was a pill that could lower the risk of chronic disease like walking does, people would be clamoring for it." One eight-year-long study of thirteen thousand people reported that subjects who walked thirty minutes per day had significantly lower risk of premature death than those who exercised rarely.

According to the National Institutes of Health (NIH), walking can:

• give you more energy and make you feel good;
• reduce stress and help you relax;
• tone your muscles;
• increase the number of calories your body uses;
• strengthen your bones and muscles;
• improve your stamina and your fitness; and
• lower your risk of chronic diseases, such as heart disease and type 2 diabetes.

No wonder Hippocrates said, "Walking is man's best medicine"!

The goal of walking ten thousand steps a day (about five miles), for example, has been suggested by many health experts, including groups like the Centers for Disease Control and Prevention and the American College of Sports Medicine. "We do have good cross-sectional studies showing that people who walk ten thousand steps per day are leaner and have lower blood pressure than those who walk less," said Professor David Bassett of the University of Tennessee on NPR's *Morning Edition* on May 16, 2005. The executive director of the President's Council on Physical Fitness, Melissa Johnson, declared, "Ten thousand steps is a phenomenal goal for people to shoot for."

These days, quite frankly, walking can be an ordeal for me, due to the effects of my MS, which can really foul up my gait and balance. Three or four blocks can be a real challenge, and a long walk for me is about a mile. Spending a day walking around at Disney World with my kids was a great victory, because I walked that whole park. It was tough, but I had to do it. Because I could be sitting around doing nothing. The heck with that!

If you're like most people and your health does allow power walking, I urge you to get moving and find any excuse you can to do it.

When you come home from work, just get out of the car and walk. Take a walk all the way down as far as you can see and come back. Then tomorrow night, go a bit farther. Grab your partner and kids and take them along too.

If you walk faster, you'll burn more calories. If you're a 150-pound woman (a man burns slightly more):

- at rest, you'll burn 60 calories an hour
- walking at 3 mph, you'll burn about 270 calories
- walking at 3.5 mph, you'll burn about 310 calories
- walking at 4 mph, you'll burn about 350 calories
- walking at 4.5 mph, you'll burn about 385 calories

Living Well Power-Walking Tips

Here are my tips and tips from the National Institutes of Health for starting your own personal walking program:

- Check with your doctor or health-care provider first, especially if you have any health issues, if you're over fifty years old and not used to doing any moderate physical activity, and if you smoke or if you are pregnant.
- Choose a safe place to walk. Find a partner or group of people to walk with you.
- Keep safety in mind when you plan your route and the time of your walk.
- If you walk at dawn, dusk, or night, wear a reflective vest or brightly colored clothing.
- Don't wear headphones.

- Wear shoes with proper arch support, a firm heel, and thick flexible soles that will cushion your feet and absorb shock.
- Think of your walk in three parts. Warm up by walking slowly for five minutes. Then, increase your speed and do a fast walk. Finally, cool down by walking slowly again for five minutes.
- Try to walk at least three times per week. Each week, add two or three minutes to your walk. If you walk less than three times per week, you may need more time to adjust before you increase the pace or frequency of your walk.
- To avoid stiff or sore muscles and joints, start gradually. Over several weeks, begin walking faster, going farther, and walking for longer periods of time.
- Keep track of your progress with a walking journal or log.
- The more you walk, the better you may feel and the more calories you may burn.
- If you can't do thirty minutes at a time, try walking for shorter amounts of time and gradually working up to it.
- Walk with your chin up and your shoulders held slightly back.
- Walk so that the heel of your foot touches the ground first. Roll your weight forward.
- Walk with your toes pointed forward.
- Swing your arms naturally as you walk.
- Also, remember that a brisk walk, which I also call a power walk, means walking fast, faster than a recreational stroll and slower than a race walk, or about three to four miles an hour.

A SAMPLE WALKING PROGRAM

WARM-UP TIME	FAST-WALK TIME	COOLDOWN TIME	TOTAL TIME
WEEK 1			
Walk slowly 5 Minutes	Walk briskly 5 Minutes	Walk slowly 5 Minutes	15 Minutes
WEEK 2			
Walk slowly 5 Minutes	Walk briskly 8 Minutes	Walk slowly 5 Minutes	18 Minutes
WEEK 3			
Walk slowly 5 Minutes	Walk briskly 11 Minutes	Walk slowly 5 Minutes	21 Minutes
WEEK 4			
Walk slowly 5 Minutes	Walk briskly 14 Minutes	Walk slowly 5 Minutes	24 Minutes
WEEK 5			
Walk slowly 5 Minutes	Walk briskly 17 Minutes	Walk slowly 5 Minutes	27 Minutes
WEEK 6			
Walk slowly 5 Minutes	Walk briskly 20 Minutes	Walk slowly 5 Minutes	30 Minutes
WEEK 7			
Walk slowly 5 Minutes	Walk briskly 23 Minutes	Walk slowly 5 Minutes	33 Minutes
WEEK 8			
Walk slowly 5 Minutes	Walk briskly 26 Minutes	Walk slowly 5 Minutes	36 Minutes
WEEK 9 and Beyond			
Walk slowly 5 Minutes	Walk briskly 30 Minutes	Walk slowly 5 Minutes	40 Minutes

If you walk less than three times per week, give yourself more than a week before increasing your pace and frequency.

Source: National Institutes of Health

LIVING WELL CHECKOFFS: DAY 10

I'll start exploring brisk walking as a way of getting regular moderate physical activity. For example, I can gradually work toward the goal of brisk walking five days a week, thirty minutes a day.

Check Here: _____

I can also shoot for the goal of walking ten thousand steps a day, or about five miles.

Check Here: _____

LIVING WELL EXPERT
Michael J. Thun, M.D.

Dr. Michael J. Thun is vice president of epidemiology and surveillance research for the American Cancer Society, one of the oldest and largest voluntary health agencies in the United States.

Dr. Thun stresses an intriguing point. While the research on diet and cancer can change over time and sometimes conflict, one pattern is becoming clear: a healthy body weight reduces your risk for cancer, and regular physical activity and a plant-based diet rich in fruits and vegetables are excellent strategies for achieving it.

Fortunately, many of the guidelines for preventing cancer are also good for preventing multiple major diseases that kill us, like heart disease and stroke and diabetes.

These guidelines are embedded in the "American Cancer Society Guidelines on Nutrition and Physical Activity and Cancer Prevention" that we published in May of 2006.

To summarize the recommendations for individuals:

Maintain a healthy weight throughout life.

- Balance caloric intake with physical activity.
- Avoid excessive weight gain throughout life.
- Achieve and maintain a healthy weight if currently overweight or obese.

Adopt a physically active lifestyle.

- Adults: Engage in at least thirty minutes of moderate-to-vigorous physical activity, above usual activities, on five or more days of the week; forty-five to sixty minutes of intentional physical activity are preferable.
- Children and adolescents: Engage in at least sixty minutes per day of moderate-to-vigorous physical activity at least five days per week.

Eat a healthy diet, with an emphasis on plant sources.

- Choose foods and beverages in amounts that help achieve and maintain a healthy weight.
- Eat five or more servings of a variety of vegetables and fruits each day.
- Choose whole grains in preference to processed (refined) grains.
- Limit consumption of processed and red meats.
- If you drink alcoholic beverages, limit consumption. Drink no more than one drink per day for women or two per day for men.

(continued)

What's distinctive about the guidelines is that two of them have moved up to the top of the list: maintaining a healthy body weight throughout your life, and being physically active.

The benefits of fruits and vegetables are much better documented for heart disease than they are for cancer. All the same time, they are an important component of maintaining a healthy body weight, because when you eat a diet that's high in fruits and vegetables it's much easier not to feel hungry all the time. And a healthy body weight reduces your risk for cancer.

I think it's pretty clear that eating fruits and vegetables is a good thing to do for health. It's a very solid recommendation, despite the limitations in the data.

We did not evolve to live in a pastry shop!

That pastry leaves you hungry for another pastry thirty minutes after you eat it. ■

LIVING WELL EXPERT
Maria Carrillo, Ph.D.

Dr. Maria Carrillo is director of medical and scientific relations for the Alzheimer's Association's National Office in Chicago.

Did you know that regular physical activity and healthy eating can reduce your risk of getting Alzheimer's disease? Dr. Carrillo has some excellent news for us.

She is responsible for overseeing the Alzheimer's Association Scientific Grant Program, and also manages its Research Roundtable, which provides a unique forum for Alzheimer's scientists from pharmaceutical companies, other companies, academia, and government to discuss trends and obstacles in Alzheimer research and therapeutic targets.

According to the Alzheimer's Association, there are now more than 5 million people in the United States living with Alzheimer's, and by 2050, the number of Americans with Alzheimer's and other dementias could soar to 16 million. The association also says that, by 2030, Alzheimer's may cost Medicare $400 billion, nearly as much as the entire current budget for Medicare.

According to Dr. Carrillo, there are simple, specific things you can start doing today that may reduce your risk for Alzheimer's. Let's you and I take charge and start putting her tips into action today.

A healthy diet and lifestyle are critical to potentially preventing or delaying the onset of Alzheimer's disease.

We know definitively that a healthy diet and a healthy lifestyle are very important to brain health. We know that the brain needs to have the right balance of nutrients, and it needs exercise, which delivers the nutrients to your brain through increased blood flow and oxygenation.

Factors that increase your risk for Alzheimer's include heart health risk factors like high blood pressure, obesity, high cholesterol, diabetes, and smoking. A long-term study of fifteen hundred adults found that those who were obese in middle age were twice as likely to develop dementia in later life. Those who also had high cholesterol and high blood pressure had six times the risk of dementia.

There are genetic risk factors for Alzheimer's, to be sure. But the whole process seems to be additive: once you have a genetic predis-

(continued)

position, these other risk factors really compound the effects and prevalence of the disease.

For example, I heard one doctor say that perhaps you're genetically predisposed to be diagnosed with Alzheimer's somewhere between age seventy-five and eighty. With the right diet and lifestyle, you could maybe push it back to between eighty and eighty-five, or even ninety, so that you never really experience the symptoms. And who wouldn't want to protect themselves for those extra years?

To protect ourselves against Alzheimer's, we need to start taking care of ourselves *now*, because Alzheimer's disease can begin in the brain ten or twenty years or more before we see symptoms on the outside.

Specifically, what can we do?

DR. CARRILLO'S TIPS:

- There's not one magic bullet, but the Alzheimer's Association recommends a well-rounded "package" of critical healthy lifestyle habits: stay physically, mentally, and socially active, and adopt a "Brain-Healthy Diet." The Alzheimer's Association calls this Maintaining Your Brain.
- Physical exercise is essential for maintaining good blood flow to the brain as well as to encourage growth of new brain cells. It also can significantly reduce the risk of heart attack, stroke, and diabetes, and thereby protect against those risk factors for Alzheimer's and other dementias.
- Growing evidence shows that physical exercise does not have to be strenuous or even require a major time commitment. It is most effective when done regularly, and in combination with a

brain-healthy diet, mental activity, and social interaction. Aerobic exercise improves oxygen consumption, which benefits brain function; aerobic fitness has been found to reduce brain cell loss in elderly subjects.

- Walking, bicycling, gardening, tai chi, yoga, and other activities of about thirty minutes daily get the body moving and the heart pumping.

- According to the most current research, a brain-healthy diet is one that reduces the risk of heart disease and diabetes, encourages good blood flow to the brain, and is low in fat and cholesterol. A brain-healthy diet is most effective when combined with physical and mental activity and social interaction. Adopt an overall food lifestyle, rather than a short-term diet, and eat in moderation.

- Reduce your intake of foods high in saturated fat and cholesterol. Studies have shown that a high intake of saturated fat and cholesterol clogs the arteries and is associated with a higher risk for Alzheimer's disease. However, HDL (or good) cholesterol may help protect brain cells, can protect you from cardiovascular risk, and can also protect you from Alzheimer's disease.

- Use mono- and polyunsaturated fats, such as olive oil. Try baking, grilling, or stir-frying food instead of deep-frying.

- Increase your intake of protective foods. Current research suggests that certain foods may reduce the risk of heart disease and stroke, and appear to protect brain cells:

  —In general, dark-skinned fruits and vegetables have the highest levels of naturally occurring antioxidants. Such vegetables include kale, spinach, Brussels sprouts, alfalfa

(continued)

sprouts, broccoli, beets, red bell pepper, onion, corn, and eggplant. Fruits with high antioxidant levels include prunes, raisins, blueberries, blackberries, strawberries, raspberries, plums, oranges, red grapes, and cherries.

—Cold-water fish contain beneficial omega-3 fatty acids: halibut, mackerel, salmon, trout, and tuna.

—Some nuts can be a useful part of your diet; almonds, pecans, and walnuts are a good source of vitamin E, an antioxidant.

—Vitamins may be helpful. There is some indication that vitamins, such as vitamin E, or vitamins E and C together, vitamin B_{12}, and folate may be important in lowering your risk of developing Alzheimer's. But there are complicating factors. For example, vitamin E supplements can negatively interact with some medications, including those prescribed to keep blood from clotting. A brain-healthy diet will help increase your intake of these vitamins and the trace elements necessary for the body to use them effectively.

Right now we don't have a way to turn back the clock, but we do know that certain lifestyle changes and good health habits may give people more time moving forward.

There is a real possibility of preventing Alzheimer's disease. We can be empowered to take control and live a much more independent life. ■

Living Well Workout: Full-Body Exercises

Not long ago, I met a guy named Bill in a business meeting.

We shook hands, and he gave me a look that's become familiar to me. When people meet me, they're really curious to see how I'm doing physically with the symptoms of MS.

Bill looked at me, smiled, and said, "Look at you—you look like solid rock!" Pointing at my chest, he added, "You could bounce bullets off that thing!"

I confess to you that I am a physical fitness nut and a gym rat, and I like being buff. Being in shape is a great feeling and it makes me more productive and energetic in everything I do. I used to spend vast periods of time in the gym. But these days, I'm so busy that I'm really concentrating on making my workouts as fast and easy as possible. Sometimes less is more, and simpler is better.

I'm at a fairly advanced level of fitness myself, but I'm constantly looking for ways to make my workouts better, more efficient, and more effective.

My workouts are a mix of the "big three" categories: aerobics (cardiovascular), resistance (strength), and flexibility (stretching). I do a good deal of stretching, and recently my workouts have gotten a bit longer because I'm holding my stretches for longer periods of time, as long as two minutes, up from the twenty to thirty seconds they used to take. As we get older we need to do a little more stretching!

In the course of a typical week, I'll alternate between two regimens:

MONTEL'S CONDENSED WORKOUT
50 minutes

- 15 minutes: aerobics/cardio; elliptical or treadmill*
- 25 minutes: strength/resistance; cables or free weights
- 10 minutes: flexibility exercises

MONTEL'S BASIC WORKOUT
90 minutes

- 25 minutes: aerobics/cardio; elliptical or treadmill*
- 45 minutes: strength/resistance; cables and free weights
- 20 minutes: flexibility exercises

For the strength-training part of my workout, I'll break my body into three muscle groups and do one group per workout: I do my chest and triceps one day; then I'll do my back and shoulders the next day, then my legs and my biceps the next day.

Now I'm going to share with you a series of easy "Intro" exercises for the next three days.

There are four groups of basic Living Well exercises: Full-Body, Upper-Body, Lower-Body, and Flexibility.

These exercises shouldn't overstress your body, and will give you something that you use as a foundation for any set of exercises you'd like to grow into.

---

*Including 5-minute warm-up and 5-minute cooldown, both at slower speeds

---

SAMPLE EXERCISE ROTATION

- Five days a week: 30-to-60-minute power walk (see Day 10)
- Each workout day: Full-Body and Flexibility Exercises
- Alternate on each workout day: either Upper-Body or Lower-Body

---

The exercises are designed to open up your body, limber up your muscles, and pump up your heart.

All you need for these exercises are:

- **a Swiss ball** (option: a beach ball, basketball, or pillow you already have)
- **exercise cables** (option: a 4- or 5-pound sand-filled exercise ball you can buy at a sporting goods shop)
- **two light dumbbells, 5 pounds each** (option: a 4- or 5-pound sand-filled exercise ball)

These exercises assume you're at a beginner's level, so we'll start with movements of short duration and gradually build up to longer ones. A few years ago I wrote a book called *BodyChange*, which includes a wide range of more advanced exercises. When you feel you're ready to move to an intermediate level, say six months from now, I suggest you check out that book. The principles in *BodyChange* are extremely sound.

The beautiful thing about exercise and physical activity is if you stick with it, it will absolutely change your life and make you feel spectacular.

Stay focused, keep moving, and be proud of yourself when you work out. Once physical activity becomes a habit, there's no feeling like it in the world. The rush you get will carry you through your toughest days and your brightest days. I've been there, and I wish for you the energy and strength to do your best.

Remember to check with your doctor first before starting these or any other exercises.

Breathing: Each time I start a workout I take about three slow, deep breaths, to pay attention to how I'm breathing and to get the blood pumping. You should remember to breathe fully throughout all your workouts.

FULL-BODY CHOP

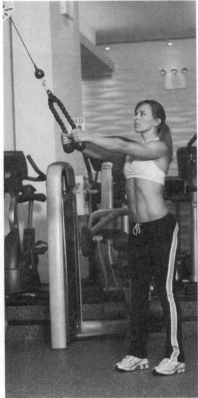

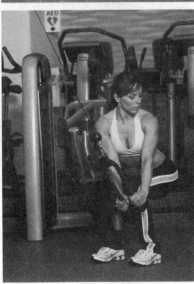

I do this exercise every other day.

Whenever you can, move your hands and arms across your heart, in a motion from side to side, or up and down; that motion is forcing your body to pump blood harder. So your heart is going to pick up its pace just a little bit, and that's the reason why I love this exercise.

If you don't have an exercise cable yet, you can replicate this motion with a household item. Just go to your cupboard and grab a one-gallon jug of water or a heavy can of sweet potatoes. Find something that's about two pounds.

- The starting position is a good straight back, arms straight, knees slightly bent, feet shoulder width apart, abs pulled in tight.
- Keeping your arms straight, pull down toward the floor in a slow, fluid, gradual motion.
- Move slowly back up to the starting position, then bring it down to the other side. That's one repetition ("rep").
- Don't twist your hips—keep them squared facing forward.
- Start with 10 repetitions.
- Over the next six weeks, work up to 12 to 15 repetitions.

REVERSE FULL-BODY CHOP

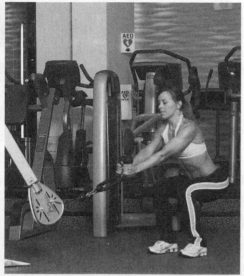

This is a great full-body exercise that incorporates every muscle from your calves, thighs, and gluteals to your obliques, abs, chest, and shoulders, all in one long motion. It's similar to the Full-Body Chop above, but in the opposite direction: your starting position is the "low" position.

With these two exercises, you work just about every single part of your body from your shoulders to your feet and ankles. They're a wonderful way to start your workout.

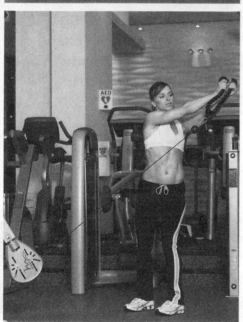

- From the starting position shown in the top photo, bring your hands up above your head, then go back down to the low starting position, then bring your arms back up to the other side, then back down to the starting position. That's one rep.
- Keep your arms straight, move in a slow, fluid, gradual motion.
- Don't twist your hips—keep them squared facing forward.
- Start with 10 repetitions.
- Over the next six weeks, work up to 12 to 15 repetitions.

FULL-BODY CROSSOVERS

This exercise works many of the key parts of the body, including "vanity areas" like the chest, pectorals, shoulders, arms, and gluteals. Our model, Wendy Traskos, who has also been a trainer for me for two years, is doing this exercise perfectly. (Note: you can check out Wendy's Web site at www.NYPoledancing.com.)

• If you don't have access to cables, just use an item like a can of peaches in each hand.

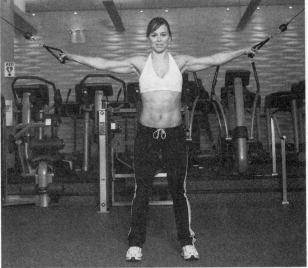

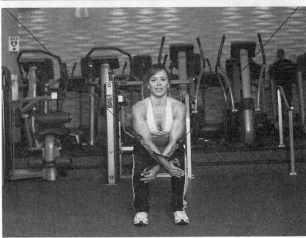

• From the starting position, move down to the crouch with your right hand over your left, then move back to the starting position. That's one rep.

• For alternate reps, cross your left hand over your right instead.

• Use a slow, fluid, gradual motion.

• Start with 10 repetitions.

• Over the next six weeks, work up to 12 to 15 repetitions.

ABDOMINAL CRUNCH

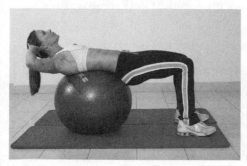 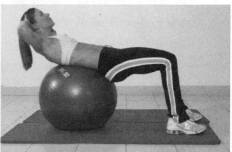

This is a great basic abdominal crunch. Doing it on a Swiss ball feels great.

The ball challenges your balance and keeps your body in proper alignment in this tabletop position. No bouncing! Make sure the ball is in the small of your back (choose the proper-sized ball to fit your height) so your body creates a tabletop position.

According to the American Council on Exercise, "Strong abdominals are key to maintaining a strong core." And while there are many different abdominal exercises, the council reports that "research suggests that abdominal crunches on a stability ball may be the most effective."

- Tabletop position: from knees to tip of head should be completely parallel with the floor when you are in starting position.
- Chin is up toward ceiling and elbows are back (not pulled up toward your face).
- Ankles should be directly under knees, and knees should be shoulder width apart, with the knees moving in the same direction as the toes.
- In the starting position of the crunch, with your body parallel to the ground, you should already feel your abs working to support this position.

- When you crunch, your body from your lower rib cage up to your head should rise only to a 35-to-45-degree angle. Don't come up to a seated position on the ball.
- Up and down is one rep.
- Start off with 10 reps, and over the next six weeks work up to 20 reps.
- This crunch can be done with your butt a little higher on the ball or a little lower on the ball. With your butt off the ball, it's easier, because the ball is going to be your support system to spring you back up. But if your butt is a little higher on the ball, the resistance is tougher.

Living Well Workout: Upper-Body Exercises

The most dangerous thing ever said in the history of physical fitness was "no pain, no gain."

When exercising, it's good to feel tension and exertion. But if it crosses the line into pain, stop right away. If you experience pain, especially sharp pain, that means your body is telling you to stop what you're doing and see a doctor.

In the gym the other day, I heard a trainer say, "This is the fastest-failing business in America." And he's absolutely right. You know why? Because if gyms worked, we wouldn't have an epidemic of obesity in America—we are the fastest-growing most obese nation on the planet!

Twenty-five years ago, the big gym craze began. Everyone started working out. Everyone hired a personal trainer. But many of them were clueless about healthy eating. That's like having a pilot who knows how to fly the right wing of the plane but doesn't know a damn thing about flying the left wing. In other words, if you want a Maserati body, you can't have a go-kart engine! You've got to fuel your body with the best Living Well foods.

Even worse, a lot of these personal trainers, unfortunately, were only skilled in working themselves out, not other people. With these guys screaming in our ears and blasting music so loud our ears bled, we overtrained, poured on the pain, hurt ourselves, and stopped working out so we could recover from the injuries. Then we put on weight from not working out, got frustrated, said "the heck with this," and stopped going to the gym. Who can blame us?

Here are five basic Upper-Body Exercises for you to enjoy, designed not for punishment or pain, but for strength, power, and Living Well.

SHOULDER PRESS

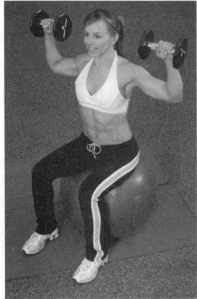

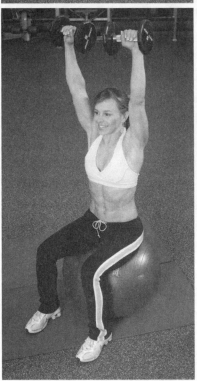

Wendy is using two light, 5-pound dumbbells here, which is a good starting weight for muscle resistance. Another option is to use a 4- or 5-pound sand-filled exercise ball.

- Start by sitting with your back straight and your stomach tight—notice how Wendy's abs are deliberately engaged and contracted.
- Using a slow, fluid, gradual motion, raise your arms up straight, then back down.
- The weights should not touch at the top of this movement—keep them more over the elbows than over the head.
- Start with 10 repetitions.
- Over the next six weeks, work up to 12 to 15 repetitions.

CHEST PRESS

I prefer free weights like these because I don't like the feeling of being tied to a weight machine. This chest press targets your pectorals, anterior deltoids, and triceps.

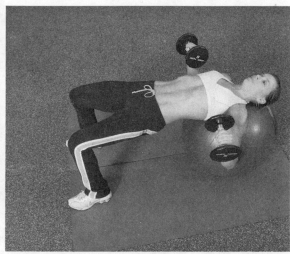

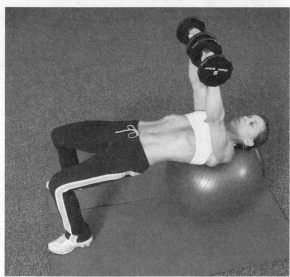

- Gently press your arms up to the point *just before* your elbows are locked in a fully extended position.
- Wait a few seconds, then move down to the starting position—be careful not to move your elbows lower than your chest level.
- You can bring the weights down *to* the chest. Just be sure you are not closing up the elbows as you lower the weights. You want to try to get full range of motion with the weights staying over your elbows, and *not* bringing them in toward the chest. This will help to stretch out the muscle as you lower, involving more muscle fibers.
- Start with 10 repetitions.
- Over the next six weeks, work up to 12 to 15 repetitions.

BACK EXERCISE

This exercise benefits your whole back. It strengthens your lower back by lifting your upper body off the floor, and with the rowing motion, you involve your upper back as well.

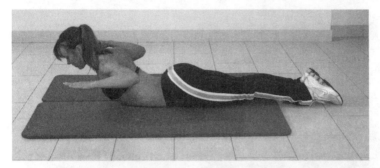

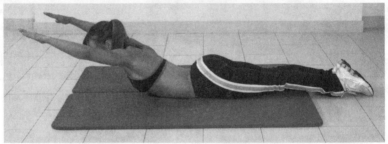

- Your lower body from your toes to your belly button should be glued to the floor.
- Lift your chest up off the floor and maintain it until you complete the exercise.
- When rowing, keep your elbows at a 90-degree angle; don't bring the hands into your shoulders.
- Hold the row contraction for just a beat, slowly coming back to the starting position.
- This is a little harder than it looks, so start off with 5 rows, and work up to 10 to 15 over the next six weeks.

BICEPS CURL

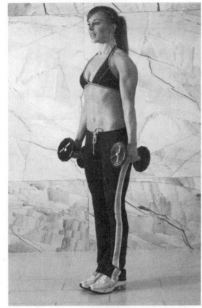

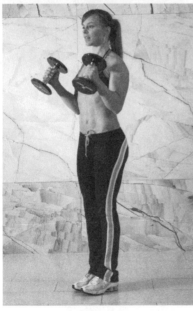

The Biceps Curl is a perfect beginning exercise. It engages the smaller muscles of your upper body, your biceps, your forearms, a little bit of your triceps, and some of your shoulder.

- Starting position: engage your abdominal muscles like Wendy is doing, with your arms hanging down.
- Slowly bring the weights up to shoulder height.
- Wait a few seconds, then slowly bring your arms down to the starting position.
- A common mistake people make: when they bring the dumbbells up to curl, they lift their elbows away from the sides of their rib cage. This is incorrect. When doing this exercise, keep your elbows right at your side.
- Start with 10 repetitions.
- Over the next six weeks, work up to 12 to 15 repetitions.

TRICEPS CURL

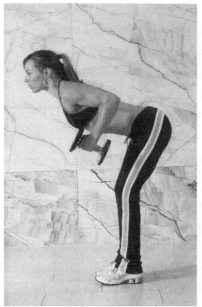

This exercise works your triceps, forearms, and a little bit of your biceps.

- From the starting position shown, while engaging your abdominals, slowly bring your arms back to be parallel with your back.
- Wait a few seconds, then gradually come back to the starting pose.
- Don't swing the weights, and keep the upper part of your arms stationary through the whole exercise.

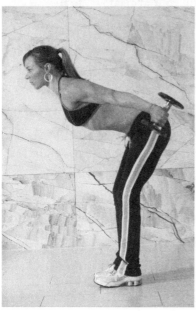

Living Well Workout: Lower-Body Exercises

SWISS BALL SQUAT

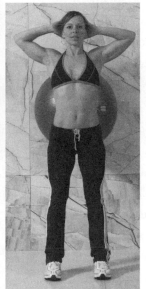

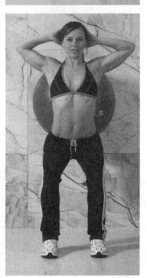

Today, let's sample three more great fundamental strength/resistance exercises; these are designed for your lower body.

This is a wonderful exercise, especially if you are a beginner. It works your core muscles, quads, hamstrings, and glutes. Using the ball, you can enjoy the benefits of a squat while your back is being supported.

- Begin with your feet shoulder width apart, with the ball against the wall and your lower back.
- As you slowly slide down, the ball supports your upper back, keeping it parallel to the wall.
- Keep your weight on your heels, as if you were sitting in a chair.
- Keep your abdominal muscles engaged, just as Wendy is doing in the picture.
- Move down until your knees are at a 90-degree angle, keeping your back pressed against the ball.
- Wait a beat, then come back up to the starting position.
- Start with 10 repetitions.
- Over the next six weeks, work up to 12 to 15 repetitions.

CALF RAISE

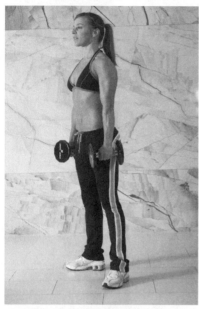

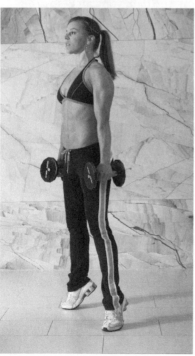

The payoff for this exercise is pretty clear: who doesn't want great-looking calves?

The calf raise strengthens the calf muscles in your lower back leg between your Achilles tendon and your knee, and helps the spring in your step when you walk, run, or bicycle. The weights help add resistance on top of your body weight, for extra strength.

- Keep your feet shoulder width apart, slightly angled out.
- Move slowly up to your tiptoes, pause a beat, and then move back down. Keep your knees and toes pointed in the same direction.
- Start with 10 repetitions.
- Over the next six weeks, work up to 12 to 15 repetitions.

HAMSTRING SWISS BALL ROLLS

Here's a wonderful move, and Wendy is doing it perfectly.

The hamstring is the key muscle on the back of your upper leg, between your butt and knee. Using the Swiss ball, this exercise works your lower body, hamstrings, back, and abs.

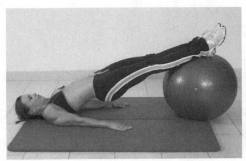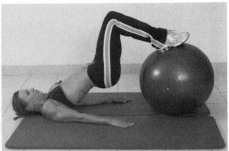

- Notice how Wendy begins by making her body a straight line from her shoulders to her feet.
- From the starting position shown, roll the ball toward you in a gradual, slow movement, hold for a beat, and then roll the ball back to the starting position. Start with 10 repetitions.
- Your hips should be as high as possible without arching your back. This will challenge your balance more and help to keep your body in proper alignment since your hips will want to drop to the floor during this exercise.
- Over the next six weeks, work up to 12 to 15 repetitions.

Living Well Workout: Flexibility Exercises

What I'm about to say is a flagrant violation of the beliefs of almost every coach and personal trainer I have ever met.

And it is contrary to what until recently my own individual beliefs were.

Here it is: don't stretch before you exercise.

For the average person doing a basic exercise or workout, it's probably an unnecessary step—and may even be a dangerous one.

Whenever you see athletes take the field, from the Miami Heat to your son's high school basketball team, you'll see them warming up on the sidelines by doing things like jogging and jumping in place. Excellent idea.

But you'll also often see them bending into deep "static" stretches, applying body weight to their extended limbs. This is probably a dumb idea, especially if it's done before the warm-up.

We've been hearing it for years in our gyms and schools: "Stretch before you exercise! It prevents injury!" Countless numbers of our kids are ordered to do this by thousands of elementary school coaches across the country every day.

Guess what—they're wrong. They've got it *backward*. It turns out that according to the latest research, there is no proof that stretching either before or after a workout reduces the risk of either muscle soreness or injury. And some studies even suggest that stretching before a workout, when muscles are cool, can actually *increase* the risk of injury.

There's a wrong way to stretch.

You see people do it in the gym all the time, or before they go running: they bounce quickly on their legs, count to ten, grab their knees and count to ten, twist their hips sharply, and bounce into another pose. Then they move on to their exercise.

That is really wrong. Stretching should not be jerking, pumping, or bouncing. The right way to stretch: relax into a stretch pose and just hold the position. You should stretch slowly and gently, and after your muscles are already warm, preferably at the end of the exercise or workout.

The consensus among many experts: stretching should be done toward the end of a workout, not before.

LIVING WELL EXPERT DISCUSSION ON STRETCHING

EXPERTS: *Ian Shrier, M.D., associate professor, department of family medicine, McGill University, Montreal, past president, Canadian Academy of Sport Medicine; and Dr. Julie Gilchrist of the U.S. Centers for Disease Control and Prevention.*

1. Is stretching a good idea, and if so, why?

DR. SHRIER: You must differentiate stretching immediately before exercise from stretching at other times. Stretching immediately before exercise does not prevent injury, and actually makes you weaker and perhaps slower. However, stretching regularly over weeks or months may prevent injuries and makes you stronger and perhaps faster.

(continued)

DR. GILCHRIST: Research in the military suggests that those who are most flexible and those who are least flexible are at increased risk of injury compared to those in the middle. Generally, people become less flexible as we age, with limited range of motion contributing to falls and other negative health outcomes in older adults. Improving flexibility and balance in the older population has been associated with improved outcomes. Thus, one might suspect that remaining somewhat flexible throughout the lifespan could be beneficial. The longitudinal study to prove this hypothesis has not been conducted. We know that those who are inflexible may be at increased injury risk and that stretching can be effective in increasing flexibility. The studies showing no benefit of pre-exercise stretching in injury prevention have all been conducted with generally athletic populations; none of the studies have controlled for participants' baseline level of flexibility. The definitive study would select two groups of relatively inflexible participants, putting one through a stretching routine over time to document increased flexibility and then comparing the resultant injury rates across groups. Unfortunately, this study has not been done.

2. Is it a better idea to stretch before or after a workout, and why?

DR. SHRIER: In general, stretching before a workout does not help, except that it acts like a painkiller. So people will feel pain relief if they are sore, but this does not mean that they are preventing injuries.

DR. GILCHRIST: Studies of stretching suggest that it is most effective in elongating muscles when the muscles are warm; thus, if one chooses to stretch, it might be most beneficial to do it during or after a workout.

3. What is the difference between a warm-up and a stretch?

DR. SHRIER: People use these terms loosely, so I guess it means whatever the person wants it to mean. For me, a stretch is when one purposefully puts the muscle through a range of motion in order to increase the range of motion. A warm-up refers to contracting and relaxing muscles in order to increase the metabolism of the muscle (this has certain advantages to performance and injury prevention).

DR. GILCHRIST: Warm-up is exactly as it sounds. To appropriately warm up, one should slowly raise the heart rate and body temperature and also move the muscles with less intensity through the anticipated range of motion (for example, a golf swing for a golfer, a light jog for a runner, etc.). Research suggests that an appropriate warm-up does decrease risk for injury.

4. Why is it that so many trainers and coaches still urge stretching before a workout—yet the latest research on the benefits is unclear or even negative?

DR. SHRIER: It takes a long time for people to change their minds about anything. This is not necessarily a bad thing when there is new evidence that contradicts old evidence—which should you believe? However, in this case, it isn't that new evidence is contradicting old evidence. Rather, there was no evidence that stretching prior to working out prevented injuries or improved performance—it was just theory that was in fact *not* grounded in basic muscle physiology.

DR. GILCHRIST: We are not sure. There are several routines in sport that continue despite evidence that they are ineffective (for example, preventively taping uninjured ankles). It may be related to the lack of scientific data in much of sport training. Thus, coaches may continue to teach what they experienced as athletes. ■

The good news is that when done properly, flexibility exercises are a key asset to your workout. According to experts at the Mayo Clinic, these exercises can improve your daily physical performance, improve the range of motion of your joints, give you better balance, help keep you mobile and less prone to injury from falls, improve circulation, maintain proper posture, lessen aches and pains, and even relieve stress.

I recently met a top exercise expert named Dr. Barbara deLateur, a professor of physical medicine and rehabilitation at Johns Hopkins University. One of the things she is very adamant about is that when you're stretching, there should be no pain at all. You should feel some tension but there should be no pain. Stretches are not supposed to hurt; they're only supposed to help your body relax.

The following exercises are designed to be held once each; in other words, they are not done in repetitions.

FULL-BODY STRETCH

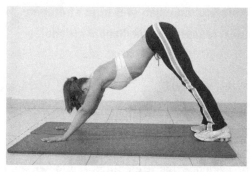

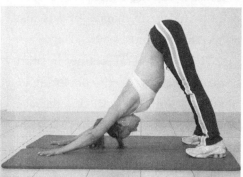

This excellent Full-Body Stretch opens up your lower spine, abdomen, hamstrings (the muscles at the back of the upper leg), glutes (gluteals, the muscles of the buttocks), and calves, all the way down to your feet.

- Hold the pose for a count of 30 seconds.
- Press your heels into the floor and aim your hips up at the ceiling.
- Get up slowly from the pose, as blood can rush to your head. If you feel dizzy, stop this pose.

- Each time you do it, try to bring your hands back a little closer to your body, with the "advanced version" as your target.
- The advanced version, the bottom photo, may take you up to six or eight weeks to achieve. It isn't exactly as easy as our fabulous trainer and model, Wendy, makes it look!

SWISS BALL STRETCH

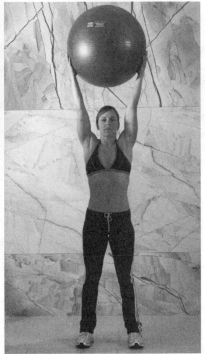

The Swiss ball is a really ingenious device. It's superlight, yet it gives you resistance. Your body reacts to the ball's unsteadiness by using more muscles to stay balanced. You can use it for lots of exercises that help build mobility, balance, and core muscle strength ("core" means back and abdominal muscles).

Many physical therapists and trainers are starting to realize that you can increase your heart rate by moving your hands from above your heart to below your heart, as we do in these poses. For some reason, these cross-body movements make your heart beat faster.

In this Swiss Ball Stretch we're loosening up our spine and building overall flexibility. If you don't have a Swiss ball yet, you can do this with a sturdy pillow, a beach ball, or a basketball.

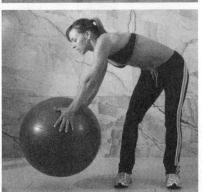

- Hold each pose for a count of 60 seconds. Over the next six weeks, work up to a goal of 2 minutes.
- Note: See how Wendy is keeping her hips squared facing forward in the second pose, not twisting her hips? That's exactly the right way to do it.

PLANK POSES

These poses are good not only for flexibility but as abdominal exercises. They're good full-body warmers. As you hold your body in these positions, you're using a good deal of core strength to keep your hips and glutes aligned.

Floor Plank

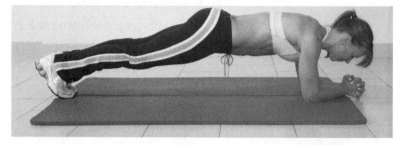

- Hold the pose for a count of 60 seconds. Over the next six weeks, work up to a goal of 2 minutes.
- Keep your elbows directly under your shoulders in a straight line.

Side Plank

- Hold the pose for a count of 60 seconds. Over the next six weeks, work up to a goal of 2 minutes.
- Repeat on the other side of your body, with your right arm on the floor.
- Keep the elbow you're leaning on in a straight line to your shoulder.

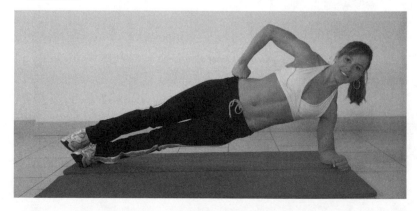

STABILITY POSES

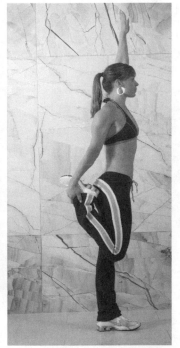

Stability poses are some of the best entry-level poses you can do. They're great for balance. I often do these moves at home or in hotels right after I wake up. I fly a lot, which can be tough on my limbs, so I'll do these exercises right on the airplane when I want to limber up.

These poses "stack" your muscles all the way from your feet to your neck. You're tightening your core muscles to hold your body rigid, so you're stretching and getting balance and stability at the same time.

Here are two basic stability poses for you to start off with. If you're an absolute beginner, you can do these near a chair or wall you can grab on to in case you lose your balance.

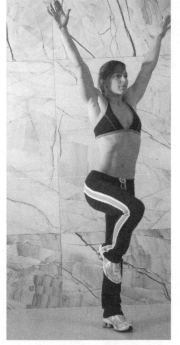

Pose 1

- Keep your body focused and still.
- Get into the pose slowly.
- Hold the pose for a count of 60 seconds. Over the next six weeks, work up to a goal of 2 minutes.
- Repeat on the reverse side—raise your left foot back, raise your right hand up.

Pose 2

- Keep your body focused and still.
- Get into the pose slowly.
- Hold the pose for a count of 60 seconds. Over the next six weeks, work up to a goal of 2 minutes.
- Repeat on the reverse side—raise your left knee.
- In the weeks ahead, gradually lengthen the time you hold the pose.

SWISS BALL BACK STRETCH

This exercise promotes flexibility in your chest, back, abs, and neck.
And it feels relaxing and terrific.

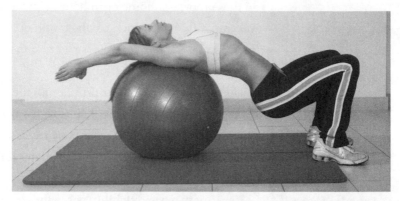

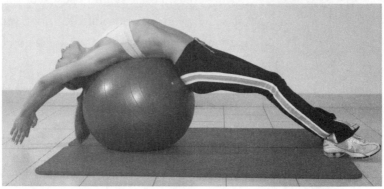

- From the starting position, slide your back gradually into the
  pose.
- Hold the pose for a count of 60 seconds. Over the next six weeks,
  work up to a goal of 2 minutes.

Live Well for Life

Small Steps:

- Start switching in healthier choices, and minimizing saturated and trans fats, sodium, processed foods, added sugars, and cholesterol from your diet.
- Start adopting healthy lifetime attitudes, like not skipping meals or going on fad diets, and building a protective home environment for your family.

LIVING WELL ACTION PLAN

WEEK 3
LIVE WELL FOR LIFE

Small Steps:
- Start switching in healthier choices, and minimizing saturated and trans fats, sodium, processed foods, added sugars, and cholesterol from your diet.
- Start adopting healthy lifetime attitudes, like not skipping meals or going on fad diets, and building a protective home environment for your family.

	MON	TUE	WED	THU	FRI	SAT	SUN
BREAKFAST							
LUNCH							
DINNER							
ALL OTHER: *Snacks, Lattes, Candy, Liquid Candy (Sugared Beverages), Office Munchies, etc.*							
PHYSICAL ACTIVITY TYPE:							
HOW MANY MINUTES:							

MY SPECIFIC PLANS TO LIVE WELL THIS WEEK:

The kinds of foods I'll enjoy:

The physical activities I'll enjoy:

The behaviors I'll make better:

The attitudes I'll make better:

Ways I'll help my family live well:

Watch the Salt

This final week of the Living Well 21-Day Program is all about Living Well for Life—by picking up some simple habits that build on what we've learned and achieved in Weeks 1 and 2 that can transform our health and make us feel spectacular.

A great place to start is with salt.

A funny thing happened to me a while ago when I gradually reduced the amount of salt in my diet.

I finally tasted my food again!

I assumed that less salt would mean less taste.

But instead the opposite was true: everything tasted better, because it tasted less like salt, and more like food.

The bad news is that by one estimate too much salt in our daily diet is killing 145,000 Americans every year. The good news is that we can start taking smart, easy steps to protect ourselves from this killer. For health purposes, salt is expressed in terms of its key ingredient, sodium. Salt is about 40 percent sodium and 60 percent chloride, so 6 grams of salt equals about 2.5 grams or 2,500 milligrams of sodium. The words "salt" and "sodium" are often used interchangeably, but keep this basic formula in mind.

One of the best things you can do to Live Well is to eat the proper amount of sodium—in other words, much less than the average American does now.

For some reason, the American food supply is overwhelmed with too much added sodium, and too much sodium raises our risk of hypertension/ high blood pressure, which in turn raises the risk of cardiovascular disease, kidney disease, and stroke.

All this sodium is literally killing us. Yet every day, the food industry keeps dumping more and more excessive amounts of salt into the food we eat.

This is a full-blown national health emergency, and thousands of people are dying every week because of it: too much sodium in our diet. The number of people who die every day from heart attacks, strokes, and other diseases caused by salt's impact on their blood pressure is equal to "a jumbo jet crashing every single day," or four hundred people, said Professor Stephen Havas of the University of Maryland School of Medicine, in the July 2005 issue of the *Nutrition Action Healthletter.* He added, "People should be outraged." I totally agree.

The situation is so dire that in 2006 the American Medical Association, representing 250,000 U.S. physicians, called on the Food and Drug Administration to revoke salt's status as a "generally recognized as safe" food ingredient, and called for a 50 percent reduction in the sodium content of processed foods, fast foods, and restaurant meals over the next ten years. The AMA has never before called for government regulation of a food ingredient.

In simple numbers, here's the problem.

The average sodium intake in the United States is about 4,000 milligrams a day. But the latest U.S. Dietary Guidelines for Americans (DGA) set a daily intake limit of sodium at 2,300 milligrams a day or less for adults up to fifty, or about a teaspoon of salt per day. Other health experts suggest an even lower maximum of 1,500 milligrams. "The relationship between salt intake and blood pressure is direct and progressive without an apparent threshold," according to the DGA, and "on average, the higher a person's salt intake, the higher is his or her blood pressure." For adults over fifty, African-Americans, and people who already have high blood pressure, the DGA recommended daily intake is 1,500 milligrams or less. Note: these are daily maximums, not recommended targets—a big difference. The body may only need 500 to 1,000 milligrams of sodium a day for general health.

Hey, no sweat, Montel, you may be thinking. *I never shake salt on my food, and I only use a pinch or two to cook with.* But you may not realize that, unfortunately, only about 10 percent of the salt we eat comes out of the salt shaker, and another 10 percent is contained naturally in foods. The whopping majority, some 75 percent, comes from processed foods, restaurant and supermarket foods.

Excessive added sodium shows up in many unexpected places, from breakfast cereal and soups to cheese and bread. "Just one cup of canned soup can contain more than 50 percent of the FDA recommended daily allowance," explained the cardiologist and American Medical Association board member Dr. J. James Rohack. "A serving of lasagna in a restaurant can put a diner over their recommended daily sodium allowance in just one meal. These examples stress the importance of a national reduction in the amount of sodium in processed and restaurant foods."

Some people believe the myth that sea salt is "better for you" than regular salt. You'll hear this in health-food stores, too, where sea salt is sold at a big price premium. But experts believe there is no nutritional difference between the two. Any extra mineral content in sea salt is nutritionally insignificant. "There is no nutritional benefit to sea salts," according to Dr. Susan Jebb, of the Medical Research Council at Cambridge University. "They all have the same amount of sodium." The big problem in America is excessive sodium consumption, not which types of salt people eat. The sales hype on sea salt may be colorful, but for health purposes, it just ain't so.

Celebrity chefs are big fans of sea salt. But the idea of using sea salt in cooking "is pure foolishness," said Robert L. Wolke, professor emeritus of chemistry at the University of Pittsburgh in the March 7, 2007, *Washington Post*, "because their sole distinction is the size and shape of their crystals, and these disappear the moment they dissolve in the food."

A huge culprit in America's salt emergency is the food and restaurant industries. Many restaurants still don't make nutritional information available on their Web sites or anywhere else, so you have no idea how much sodium you're eating. I call this invisible salt. Food manufacturers are still flooding much of our food with sodium, but at least in most cases they're required by law to print the sodium content on the package, so I call this stealth salt.

Take a look at these shocking stats:

EXAMPLES OF STEALTH AND INVISIBLE SODIUM IN COMMON FOODS

- The American Medical Association says: 480 milligrams of sodium per serving is "high in salt."
- Most experts set 1,500 to 2,400 milligrams as a daily adult maximum.

Food	Sodium per Serving (milligrams)
General Tso's chicken (Chinese restaurant)	3,200
Combination fried rice (Chinese restaurant)	2,700
Hungry-Man XXL Roasted Carved Turkey frozen dinner	2,240*
Bertolli Italian Sausage & Rigatoni frozen dinner	1,360
Nissin Cup Noodles Beef Flavor Ramen Noodles	1,110
Starbucks Tarragon Chicken Salad sandwich	1,100
Muir Glen Organic Soup, Classic Minestrone	960*
South Beach Diet Frozen Beef & Broccoli with Asian Style Noodles	950
Progresso Chicken Noodle Soup	950*
Campbell's Select Beef Stock Minestrone	900*
Kids Cuisine frozen Mac and Cheese	750
Knorr-Lipton Chicken Pasta Sides mix with Whole Grains	810
NutriSystem packaged pizza	780

*A container contains 2 servings, so if you eat the whole thing, double the sodium number.
Source: Chinese restaurant items: Center for Science in the Public Interest; others: author store checks.

By reducing your sodium consumption to the recommended levels, you'll be doing your health a big favor. A major study published in the April 2007 issue of the *British Medical Journal* demonstrated that "lowering sodium can reduce the risk of later cardiovascular disease, even among people with hypertension," according to study researcher Dr. Nancy Cook of Harvard Medical School.

Living Well Tips on Sodium: 10 Positive Steps You Can Take Right Now

1. See your doctor and have your blood pressure checked ASAP. Talk these tips over with him or her.
2. Rather than suddenly slashing your sodium intake, try reducing it gradually over a few weeks. You may not even notice the difference, and if you're like me, you won't miss it at all.
3. Keep an eye on Nutrition Facts labels, and shoot for a daily sodium consumption of less than 2,300 milligrams of sodium per day, or better yet, less than 1,500 per day. If you're over fifty, an African-American, or have high blood pressure, shoot for less than 1,500 milligrams of sodium per day.
4. Remember that foods with more than 480 milligrams of sodium per serving are considered high in salt.
5. Instead of table salt, use sodium-free or low-sodium seasonings like herbs, pepper, spices, lemon, lime, garlic, salt-free seasoning blends, and herbs.
6. Double-check the serving size on the Nutrition Facts labels: soup, for example, often comes in two-serving cans, meaning you have to double the numbers if you eat it all yourself.
7. Select foods without added salt whenever you can. Limit the amount of salty snacks you eat, like chips and pretzels.
8. Eat fewer processed foods—including take-out, ready-to-eat, prepared, and fast food—and more fresh foods, like whole fruits and vegetables, whole grains, and fish; and if you're into lean meat and poultry, make it unsalted.
9. Look into the DASH Diet. It's an eating plan developed by leading scientists, doctors, and the National Institutes of Health that can lead to significant, rapid reductions in blood pressure, on par with single-drug therapy in individuals with mild hypertension. For a

free sixty-four-page online book, *The DASH Eating Plan*, go to the resources section at the end of this book.

10. Beef up on potassium: potassium counteracts some of sodium's effects on blood pressure. Potassium-rich foods include sweet potatoes, orange juice, bananas, spinach, winter squash, cantaloupe, tomato puree, beets, broccoli, and tomatoes. The Institute of Medicine suggests a potassium intake for adults of 4,700 milligrams per day, which is about 40 percent more than the average American gets.

LIVING WELL CHECKOFFS: DAY 15

I'll make an appointment today with my health-care provider to check my blood pressure, which is a major risk factor for cardiovascular disease.

Check Here: _____

Starting today, I'll pay attention to my sodium intake, and over the next few weeks I'll start gradually reducing it to a healthy adult range of less than 2,300 milligrams per day, and less than 1,500 per day if I'm over fifty, African-American, or have high blood pressure.

Check Here: _____

Instead of adding lots of salt to my foods and cooking, I'll start enjoying herbs, pepper, spices, lemon, lime, garlic, and salt-free seasonings instead.

Check Here: _____

Be a Portion Controller

You know what?

I can pull up my shirt right now and show you my six-pack.

A big reason for this, beyond my exercise and healthy food choices, is that I eat food portions fit for humans, not the Gigantor-sized monstrosities we have been cursed with in America.

We live in a society where everything has to come in a supersize. When we go to a restaurant, if we don't see our plates full we feel we're being ripped off. But the truth is that the average American is eating roughly 30 percent more daily calories than necessary, and it's all adding up to make us sick.

Even the manufacturers of household dishware have caught on to supersizing. At home, you may be eating on a dish that's twelve or thirteen inches wide. That's not a plate—it's a platter!

When it comes to food, I have a pretty simple rule: I eat until I'm not hungry. I eat to feel good, not to gorge myself. I think the all-American all-you-can-eat buffet is one of the dumbest ideas ever! I don't pile big portions on my plate and figure I have to eat it all. I eat moderate portions, and I enjoy every bite. When I'm done eating, I feel good. I push the plate away; then I get up and walk away.

Sometimes I eat five meals a day, sometimes six, and sometimes three or four. I eat everything I want, and I am telling you, I don't feel deprived at all.

It is time you and I declared war on belly-busting food portions.

Research shows that the more food you put in front of you, and the bigger the portions are, the more you'll eat. You'll stuff yourself without realizing it. The result: we have a nation of children and adults waddling around the United States in stretch pants with jumbo potbellies and butts so big they can barely fit in an airplane seat! And it's no laughing matter—obesity is a dangerous, debilitating, life-threatening illness.

We have fallen victim to what I call Creeping Portion Madness.

We continue to suffer from an epidemic of Big Gulps, Supersizes, and Grand Slam breakfasts. Our kids now look at a mountain of food dumped on a plate or a gargantuan serving of dessert and figure it's a normal way to eat. Over the last twenty to thirty years, restaurants and food companies have gradually doubled many of our standard portion sizes. Here are just a few examples:

Living Badly: Creeping Portion Madness in America

	Portion size in calories	
	20 years ago	**Today**
Blueberry muffin	210	500
Cheeseburger	333	590
French fries	210	610
Spaghetti and meatballs	500	1,025
Turkey sandwich	320	820
Soda	85	250
Chicken Caesar salad	390	790
Bagel	140	350
Popcorn	210	630
Cheesecake	260	640
Chocolate-chip cookie	55	275

Source: National Heart, Lung and Blood Institute.

LIVING WELL: THE CORRECT SERVING SIZES

MEAT AND FISH

This is surprising, and really important: the correct standard serving size of a piece of meat is only the size of a deck of cards, not the enormous serving sizes of steak and beef we've gotten used to.

1 Serving Size Looks Like . . .

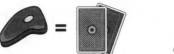

3 ounces fish, lean meat, or poultry = a deck of cards

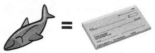

3 ounces grilled/baked fish = a checkbook

GRAIN PRODUCTS

If you're a pasta lover, how's this for a bombshell: the correct standard serving size for a half cup of cooked pasta is only about the size of half a baseball! If you routinely eat jumbo restaurant pasta portions, you're consuming a heck of a lot of extra calories.

1 Serving Size Looks Like . . .

1 slice of bread = a cassette tape

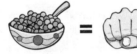

1 cup of cereal flakes = the size of your fist

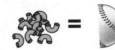

½ cup of cooked rice or pasta = ½ baseball

VEGETABLES AND FRUIT

Now here's something really interesting: many health experts and authorities recommend we eat between five and thirteen servings of fruits, and vegetables, or even more, per day, which seems like an enormous amount! But it's less than you might imagine. Roughly speaking, a serving of fruit or vegetables is the amount that would fit in the palm of your hand. A big salad can easily account for three veggie servings.

1 Serving Size Looks Like . . .

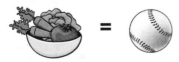

1 cup of raw veggies = a baseball, or a woman's fist
1 cup of salad greens = a baseball, or a woman's fist

½ cup of cooked veggies or beans = ½ baseball
½ cup of fresh fruit = ½ baseball

Isn't this amazing? No wonder we've gotten so fat and sick! Americans are routinely stuffing down 1,000 or 2,000 calories a day more than they should to maintain a healthy body weight. The weird thing is, I don't remember anybody twenty years ago saying that portion sizes were too small and that we simply had to have bigger portions. It just happened.

The portion sizes that you've gotten used to eating could easily be equal to double the standard serving size, and therefore double the calories, saturated fat, and sodium listed for a standard serving. To Live Well, we've got to get back to eating the proper serving sizes.

Fruits and veggies are the one thing I'd suggest you not worry about when it comes to portion control, as long as you're eating them without added salt, sodium, or other extras: your motto should be "more is better."

The New Living Well Plate

Let's do a gentle, beautiful makeover of your dinner plate.

I don't want you to restrict your diet.

I want you to correct the way you look at the proportions of food on the plate, so you'll get fuller and healthier on fewer calories.

I call it the New Living Well Plate. It is directly inspired by a fantastic concept from the experts at the American Institute for Cancer Research (AICR) called the New American Plate. They suggest that instead of trying to count every single calorie we eat, we simply "make over" our plate. Instead of the traditional plate divided into one-half meat, one-quarter potatoes, and one-quarter vegetable, we should make our meat portion smaller, with the extra space going to more vegetables, fruits, whole grains, and beans.

Sources for page 214: National Heart, Lung and Blood Institute; American Dietetic Association, American Cancer Society. FYI: What's the difference between a portion and a serving? A "portion" is how much food you choose to eat, whether in a restaurant, from a package, or in your kitchen. A "serving" is a standard amount set by the U.S. government.

BORING OLD AMERICAN MEAL

6 ounces meat over half of plate

overcooked carrots

On the side:

a white roll and butter

salt shaker

small mixed green salad

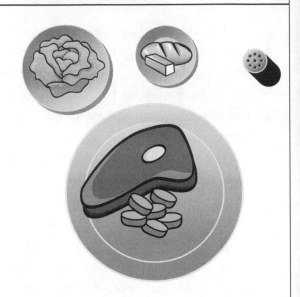

THE *NEW* LIVING WELL AMERICAN MEAL

3 ounces fish or lean meat
(the size of a deck of cards)
one-third of plate

sliced microwaved sweet potato

kidney beans

On the side:

bowl of low-sodium vegetable soup

big bowl of mixed greens salad seasoned
with herbs and extra-virgin olive oil

1/2 cup brown rice
(from ninety second microwave pouch)

shaker of herbs

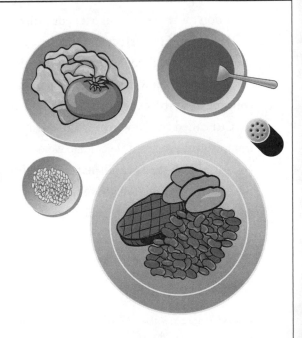

"We're talking about shifting the traditional meal around a bit," says AICR nutrition adviser Karen Collins, R.D., "so that at least two-thirds of the plate contains the kind of plant-based foods that actively fight chronic disease, while one-third or less contains meat, poultry, or fish."

LIVING WELL CHECKOFF: DAY 16

Starting today, I'm going to start saying yes to sensible portion sizes, and to more vegetables, fruits, whole grains, and beans on my plate.

Check Here: _____

LIVING WELL EXPERT
Ann Albright, Ph.D., R.D.

Dr. Ann Albright is president, Health Care and Education for the American Diabetes Association.

The American Diabetes Association is the leading nonprofit health organization dedicated to preventing and curing diabetes. Albright has also served as the senior health policy adviser for the Office of the U.S. Surgeon General.

I've been connected to diabetes for a long time, not just professionally but personally—I've lived with type 1 diabetes for forty years.

People don't realize that diabetes is the number-one cause of adult blindness in this country. It's the number-one cause of nontraumatic lower limb amputation. It's the number-one cause of kidney failure in the country. And it's a huge contributor to heart diseases and stroke, the foremost causes of death in this country.

(continued)

Right now, there are about 21 million people with diabetes, about 90 to 95 percent of them with type 2 diabetes. There are another 54 million with prediabetes. Type 2 diabetes is not inevitable. Many people think, *Well, I'm genetically predisposed, it doesn't matter what I do, it's going to happen to me anyway.* Diabetes is so pervasive in some cultures that people think, *Everybody I know has diabetes and so will I.*

It's not inevitable!

Another misconception is that eating sugar causes diabetes. That's not the case. Type 1 diabetes is the result of a genetic malfunction. Type 2 diabetes is most often the result of a genetic predisposition combined with unhealthy lifestyle habits. Elliot Joslin described type 2 diabetes this way: Your genes load the cannon, and your diet and lifestyle light the fuse.

We can't yet prevent type 1 diabetes, but type 2 is preventable, or at least can be postponed, and your diet and physical activity can be even more effective than the medication you need to take.

The first step is to understand what healthy food choices are. I strongly encourage people to talk to a registered dietitian to put together a nutrition plan that's specifically designed for the individual and their medical situation. Diabetics must maintain a healthy weight. It's important to pay attention to your carbohydrate intake. This doesn't mean you need to eat a low-carb diet. Your carbohydrates should be rich in fiber, and you should be eating plenty of nonstarchy vegetables and fruit. Eat fish two or three times a week. Your meat and poultry should be the lean cuts and your dairy should be no-fat and low-fat.

To reduce the risk of type 2 diabetes the best lifestyle tip is to lose weight if necessary and be as active as you can—thirty minutes of physical activity most days of the week. You don't have to do it all at one time. Take the steps instead of elevators and escalators. Park your car at the far end of the parking lot and walk to the store. Ride a bike or take a long walk. Carve out time in your schedule for physical activity, particularly if you're trying to lose weight and then to maintain the weight loss, because you may really need more than thirty minutes of physical activity a day for weight-loss maintenance. Physical activity is critical not only for maintenance of weight loss and prevention of type 2 diabetes, but also for managing diabetes.

Many people think, *Hey, I'm too busy. That's too much work.* Or *Oh my gosh, thirty minutes of physical activity a day? There is no way I can do that!* But on Day 1, maybe it's just getting some good walking shoes or exercise shoes out of your closet and walking around the block. You need to start where you are. Just get started. Try to do something and then build on it. There really is no downside to being physically active.

The average American diet today is like a burning building. It is increasing our risk for type 2 diabetes, heart disease, high blood pressure, cancer, and other diseases. Why would you stay in a burning building? If you don't have your health, you really can't enjoy much of anything else in life.

People with diabetes are a very high risk for heart attack. We give a lot of attention to the carbohydrate intake, but we've got to also pay attention to saturated fat and its negative consequences. And that's another reason for people to eat more fresh fruits and vegetables, and low-fat protein sources: to minimize saturated fat in their diet.

This is a good-news story. Diabetes can have devastating consequences, but with the better tools and better information we have now, you can do your very best to stack the deck in your favor.

If you improve your diet and lifestyle, take medication as prescribed, and work with medical professionals to help you cope with and adjust your diabetes treatment plan, you will give yourself the best possible opportunity to have a healthy life.

(continued)

Here are some tips from the American Diabetes Association for making healthful food choices for you and your entire family.

- Eat lots of vegetables and fruits. Try picking from the rainbow of colors available to maximize variety. Eat nonstarchy vegetables, such as spinach, carrots, broccoli, or green beans with meals.
- Choose whole-grain foods over processed grain products. Try brown rice with your stir-fry or whole wheat spaghetti with your favorite pasta sauce.
- Include dried beans (like kidney or pinto beans) and lentils in your meals.
- Include fish in your meals two to three times a week.
- Choose lean meats like cuts of beef and pork that end in "loin," such as pork loin and sirloin. Remove the skin from chicken and turkey.
- Choose nonfat dairy, such as skim milk, nonfat yogurt, and non-fat cheese.
- Choose water and calorie-free "diet" drinks instead of regular soda, fruit punch, sweet tea, and other sugar-sweetened drinks.
- Choose liquid oils for cooking instead of solid fats that can be high in saturated and trans fats. Remember that fats are high in calories. If you're trying to lose weight, watch your portion sizes of added fats.
- Cut back on high-calorie snack foods and desserts like chips, cookies, cakes, and full-fat ice cream.
- Eating too much of even healthful foods can lead to weight gain. Watch your portion sizes.

The more you commit to healthy living and the more you build on it, the more you'll reap the benefits, like Montel has. He feels so much better when he is eating healthfully and active physically, and so will you. ■

Be a Label Sleuth

You should see me when I'm set loose in a grocery store.

I am a flat-out label sleuth.

When I'm food shopping, I always flip the packages over and check out the nutrition stats on the Nutrition Facts label. I'm grabbing and flipping, eyeballing the stats, and lots of times I'm tossing the packages right back on the shelf—too much saturated fat, too much sodium, not enough vitamin C.

I am one picky son of a gun. You should be, too!

Wait a minute. Maybe you're thinking, *C'mon, Montel, get real! Those labels are confusing! How am I supposed to do the math? You think I've got time to shop with a slide rule and a calculator? Forget it!*

I've got two thoughts for you.

First, don't be afraid. Don't zone out at the numbers and percentages. It's not that hard at all when you know how to "cheat" a little. I've even prepared a cheat sheet you can take with you to the store.

Second, this is supercritical information for you and your family's health.

It's like checking under the hood and kicking the tires when you're buying a car, or checking out the diplomas on a doctor's wall, or looking in the closets when you buy a house. I'm serious!

The stuff we put in our bodies is absolutely no less important—it can kill us or it can make us healthy. Plus, we're paying darn good hard-earned money to the food companies, and we've got to pay attention to this critical information.

First I check to make sure the ingredient list doesn't contain a long list of nasty-sounding ingredients that sound like they came out of Dr. Frankenstein's lab. My theory is, the shorter the ingredient list, the better it is for me.

Then I scan some of the key numbers on the Nutrition Facts label.

I do this all the time with packaged food, even if it claims to be a health food and there are colorful splashy banners and dancing cartoons on the package that shout "Now Made With Whole Grains!" or "Zero Cholesterol and Zero Trans Fat!"

Well, that's nice, but I'm extraskeptical about this kind of sales puffery, since sometimes it's a tactic used by the manufacturer to divert your attention from facts like the food is low in nutrients or fiber, or high in sodium.

I was in the health-food store the other day and I saw a box on the shelf that read "healthy granola." I flipped it over and saw that it had so many weird, funky-looking ingredients it looked like a chemical factory!

How to Be a Label Sleuth by Being Label Aware

I suggest you be "label aware," not "label obsessed." That means sticking a copy of the cheat sheet on the next page in your purse or wallet and referring to it when you shop. Keep rough, running totals in your mind for things like calories, saturated and trans fats, and sodium.

You can't do this with everything: some food items, like produce, don't yet require nutrition labeling, but it's hard to go wrong nutritionally with a variety of fruits and vegetables.

THE LIVING WELL NUTRITION FACTS CHEAT SHEET

Nutrition Facts

Serving Size 1 cup (228g)
Servings Per Container 2

Amount Per Serving	
Calories 250	Calories from Fat 110

	% Daily Value*
Total Fat 12g	18%
Saturated Fat 3g	15%
Trans Fat 1.5g	
Cholesterol 30mg	10%
Sodium 470mg	20%
Total Carbohydrate 31g	10%
Dietary Fiber 0g	0%
Sugars 5g	
Protein 5g	
Vitamin A	4%
Vitamin C	2%
Calcium	20%
Iron	4%

*Percent Daily Values are based on a 2,000 calorie diet.
Your Daily Values may be higher or lower depending on
your calorie needs:

	Calories:	2,000	2,500
Total Fat	Less than	65g	80g
Sat Fat	Less than	20g	25g
Cholesterol	Less than	300mg	300mg
Sodium	Less than	2,400mg	2,400mg
Total Carbohydrate		300g	375g
Dietary Fiber		25g	30g

Servings per container: Check the serving size and number of servings. The label information is based on one serving, but many packages contain more. If you double the servings you eat, you double the calories and nutrients, including the percent DVs.

Calories: Calories count, so pay attention to the amount. Fat-free doesn't mean calorie-free. Lower-fat items may have as many calories as full-fat versions.

Total Fat: Eat less than 65 grams per day. To help lower blood cholesterol, replace saturated and trans fats with monounsaturated and polyunsaturated fats found in fish, nuts, and liquid vegetable oils, such as corn, safflower, sunflower, olive, and canola oils. Most fats should come from these types of sources of polyunsaturated and monounsaturated fats.

Saturated Fat: Eat less than 20 grams per day. The major way to keep saturated fat low is to limit your intake of animal fats, like those in full-fat dairy products (cheese, milk, butter, ice cream); fatty meat; bacon and sausage; and poultry skin and fat.

Trans Fat: Eat zero or as little as possible. The major way to limit trans fat intake is to limit the intake of foods made with partially hydrogenated vegetable oils.

Cholesterol: Keep under 300 milligrams per day, some experts suggest under 200 milligrams.

Sodium: Over 480 milligrams per serving is considered high in sodium. Keep your total under 2,300 milligrams per day (under 1,500 milligrams per day may be better yet), or under 1,500 milligrams a day if you are over fifty, or are African-American, or have high blood pressure.

Potassium: Experts recommend at least 3,500 milligrams to 4,700 milligrams per day.

Total Carbohydrate: You want to favor healthy carbohydrates from sources like fruits, vegetables, beans, and whole grains. Fiber and sugars are types of carbohydrates.

Dietary Fiber: Aim for a daily intake of 25 to 30 grams, from sources like whole grains, fruits and vegetables, and beans.

Sugars: There isn't a percent DV for sugar, but you can compare the sugar content in grams among products.

Protein: Protein intake is not a public health concern for adults and children over four years of age. Most Americans get plenty of protein, but not always from the healthiest sources. When choosing a food for its protein content, such as meat, poultry, milk, and milk products, make choices that are lean, low-fat, or fat-free.

Vitamin A, Vitamin C, Calcium, Iron: Look for different foods that are rich in these nutrients.

Sources: FDA Center for Food Safety and Applied Nutrition, Dietary Guidelines for Americans, Institutes of Medicine, American Heart Association, author's research.

Rules of Thumb:

- Keep low: saturated fat, trans fat, cholesterol, and sodium.
- Keep high: fiber, potassium, iron, calcium, and vitamins A and C.
- The general rule of thumb is that 5 percent or less of the Daily Value is considered low and 20 percent or more is high.
- Choose the most nutritionally rich foods you can from each food group each day—those packed with vitamins, minerals, fiber, and other nutrients but lower in calories.
- Check the ingredients list, and limit foods with added sugars (sucrose, glucose, fructose, corn, or maple syrup), which add calories but not other nutrients, such as vitamins and minerals. Make sure that added sugars are not one of the first few items in the ingredients list.
- Whole-grain foods can't always be identified by color or name, such as multigrain or wheat. Look for the "whole" grain listed first in the ingredient list, such as whole wheat, brown rice, or whole oats.
- These tips are general rules of thumb for adults. Different values may apply for children, women of childbearing age, the elderly, and other groups. The percent DV is based on a 2,000-calorie diet. You may need more or less, but the percent DV is still a helpful gauge.

LIVING WELL CHECKOFF: DAY 17

I will start paying attention to Nutrition Facts labels, to keep my overall intake of saturated fat, trans fat, cholesterol, and sodium low—and nutrients like fiber, potassium, iron, calcium, and vitamins A and C high.

Check Here: _____

LIVING WELL SPOTLIGHT
Neurodegenerative Diseases Like Parkinson's Disease and Multiple Sclerosis

Unlike heart disease and obesity, neurodegenerative diseases like multiple sclerosis (MS), Parkinson's disease (PD), and amyotrophic lateral sclerosis (ALS, also known as Lou Gehrig's disease) are not yet known to be caused or strongly influenced by a person's diet. In fact, last year a group of experts wrote that "no nutritional agent has to date been shown to have the capacity to alter the course of any neurodegenerative disease."

But at the same time, it may be extra-important for people facing these health challenges to follow the patterns of the Living Well Code, after consulting with their doctor. For example, the National Parkinson Foundation says that while nutrition won't cure PD or slow its progression, "nutrition does indeed make a significant contribution to the health status of persons living with Parkinson's disease." Here's what some top experts say about Living Well with neurodegenerative diseases.

Kathrynne Holden is a registered dietitian (R.D.) and leading authority in nutrition, dietary needs, and complementary treatments for Parkinson's disease. She has pioneered understanding of the nutrition concerns that occur with PD, and works to prevent nutrition-related hospitalizations, make the best use of medications, and maintain an independent lifestyle.

Holden is the author of Eat Well, Stay Well with Parkinson's Disease *and* Cook Well, Stay Well with Parkinson's Disease, *and she hosts the "Ask the Parkinson Dietitian" forum on www.parkinson.org, the Web site of the National Parkinson Foundation.*

(continued)

As far as I know, I am the only dietitian specializing in Parkinson's disease (PD). There are fewer people with PD than, say, diabetes or cancer, and in many places, too few patients for local dietitians to be able to focus on PD alone. So PD doesn't receive the attention, the focus, or the research funding, including research into nutritional concerns. The result is that there's a lot we just don't know.

Regarding diet to prevent PD, I would love to say, "If you eat healthful foods and don't eat saturated fat, it's going to lower your risk for Parkinson's." But the research isn't there, so it's never been proven. I think it's highly possible, but without research there is no proof.

There appears to be an association with dietary vitamin E and lowered risk of Parkinson's. There also appears to be an association between coffee consumption and regular exercise and lowered risk of Parkinson's.

I think it's possible that there could be a link between vitamin D deficiency and PD. This is speculation, purely from my own observations. However, this deficiency has recently been linked to cancer, metabolic syndrome, high blood pressure, autoimmune diseases, multiple sclerosis, and diabetes (and, possibly of significance, there is a suggestion that diabetes itself increases risk for PD). I would like to see research conducted in this area. In the meantime, vitamin D is certainly a factor in many diseases, and I encourage people to get enough vitamin D in their diet, whether they have PD or not.

We also need more research on B vitamins. There was a small study on PD done in Brazil. Out of thirty subjects with PD, the researchers found that every single one of them was deficient in riboflavin, a B vitamin. They gave the subjects supplements of riboflavin and omitted red meat from their diet, and every patient showed some amelioration of Parkinson's symptoms. It was a very small study; you can't draw any conclusions from it, and unfortunately no one has done any further work on it. But B vitamins come up over and over in regard to PD.

Another study suggested that people who got the most vitamin E from food in their diets (not from supplements) had a lower risk of PD. I thought that was fairly interesting. Vitamin E is a powerful antioxidant, and it's possible that it could be protective against PD in some way.

But apart from that, prudence dictates that antioxidants should be a good thing for someone who suffers from free radical damage. Parkinson's is an extremely stressful disease, and stress creates free radicals. Antioxidants combat free radical damage from the stress. I encourage people to eat walnuts, almonds, peanut butter, sunflower seeds, and other sources of dietary vitamin E, whether vitamin E prevents PD or not.

There is a very high incidence of depression in Parkinson's disease, and it is not always managed by antidepressants. It's pretty well established that omega-3 fatty acids alleviate certain forms of depression that have not been managed by antidepressants. I don't know of any research done on omega-3 fatty acids for PD, but due to the high incidence of depression, and the fact that it's not always alleviated by antidepressants, I encourage people with Parkinson's to eat fish or take omega-3 supplements.

Parkinson's can be debilitating in every conceivable way. It's a progressive, incurable disease that manages to cover the entire spectrum of risk factors for malnutrition. It can slow movement of the gastrointestinal tract, resulting in constipation, slowed stomach emptying, and choking. Medications can cause nausea, appetite loss, and weight loss. As Parkinson's progresses, there can be bowel impaction, inability to manage eating utensils, increased risk for falls and bone fractures, and yet less ability to eat food that contains the vitamins and minerals that keep bones and muscles strong.

(continued)

Nevertheless, with attention to diet, people with PD can prevent nutrition-related diseases and hospitalizations. If ever there was a population that desperately needed an optimal diet—high in vegetables, fruits, fish, and whole grains—it's people with Parkinson's disease. Good nutrition is a major factor in maintaining the best possible overall physical and mental health.

* * *

Alberto Ascherio, M.D., Ph.D., is associate professor of nutrition and epidemiology at the Harvard University School of Public Health.

His research focuses on identifying causes, risk factors (positive and negative), prevention, and early detection of multiple sclerosis (MS), Parkinson's disease (PD), and amyotrophic lateral sclerosis (ALS, also known as Lou Gehrig's disease).

Dr. Ascherio stresses that we just don't have a great deal of knowledge yet in these fields—but he identifies some of the promising developments that may lie just over the horizon.

With PD and ALS, the long-standing hypothesis has been that oxidative stress plays a role in these diseases. If you look at the brains of people who died of PD and ALS, it seems pretty clear that there was oxidative stress, and we know that diet contributes important antioxidants. But so far, the attempts to link dietary antioxidants to the risk of developing PD or ALS have not produced really convincing results.

In the case of ALS, the hypothesis that major antioxidants like vitamin E could be protective has been around for many years, and in fact we found in one study that high doses of vitamin E were related study. We're working to confirm this preliminary result with a five-year grant from the National Institutes of Health. In animal models, vitamin E seems to provide some benefit, but in humans the results were disappointing in terms of treatment. So whether dietary vitamin E or other antioxidants may reduce the risk of ALS is a hope at this stage, but we don't have definitive data.

For PD, an emerging and promising finding is that high levels of urate in plasma are associated with a lower risk of developing Parkinson's and slower disease progression. Urate is a potent antioxidant, and a beneficial effect of urate fits well with the hypothesis that oxidative stress is important in PD. Urate levels can be increased by taking dietary supplements of inosine. Although high levels of urate are related to the metabolic syndrome (a group of medical disorders that increase risk for cardiovascular disease and diabetes) and higher risk of gout and cardiovascular disease and hypertension, in individuals with Parkinson's disease or at high risk of Parkinson's disease, a moderate elevation of urate could be beneficial. Attempts to increase urate levels to slow the progression of PD, however, should for now be pursued only in carefully monitored and rigorously controlled clinical trials, because of the uncertain efficacy and potential adverse effects.

Probably the most promising data are on multiple sclerosis (MS). Multiple sclerosis is a neurological disease with a strong autoimmune component and possible infectious triggers. There is accumulating evidence that vitamin D, not only from diet but from sunlight exposure, is associated with a lower risk of developing MS.

In latitudes like Boston, where I live, most people go through a period of vitamin D deficiency during the winter. Unless you take high doses of supplements, your vitamin D level will dip below the optimal level, and the evidence is accumulating that this vitamin D deficiency

(continued)

may markedly increase the risk of MS. The strongest association is found in people who are eighteen to twenty years old. By giving vitamin D supplements to this age group, it may be possible to reduce the incidence of MS by a half.

In the field of diet and neurological diseases, this is the most promising and exciting finding. The problem is that we need a large experiment, a large randomized trial, to see if giving kids vitamin D supplements will prevent them from getting MS. Some researchers think we should just start giving out the vitamin D, whereas others don't believe that available evidence supports a causal effect. Thirty years from now, we'll probably still be debating, unless we do a large trial soon.

For people who are at higher risk of MS because of their family history, it's not unreasonable to think about supplementing with vitamin D, especially when you consider that vitamin D, in the amount proposed to prevent MS, is extremely safe and likely to be beneficial to prevent other diseases, such as osteoporosis.

Overall, with few exceptions, the connections between diet and neurological diseases are still largely unknown, and it is thus too early to make specific dietary recommendations. This is an exciting and rapidly moving field, however, and we should all stay posted for further news.

* * *

Noel R. Rose, M.D., Ph.D., is director of the Center for Autoimmune Disease Research at Johns Hopkins University and served as chairman of a committee to coordinate research studies into autoimmune disease at the National Institutes of Health.

He is an expert in autoimmunity, which is a major cause of human disease. In the United States, 15 to 22 million people suffer from autoimmune diseases, which include type 1 diabetes, multiple sclerosis, lupus, celiac disease, Crohn's disease, and rheumatoid arthritis, among many others.

While there's a lot we don't know yet, Dr. Rose tells us what we can do to keep our immune system in fighting shape.

A well-balanced diet combined with exercise is the best way to keep a healthy immune system.

Most scientists feel that autoimmune disease is a consequence of an interaction between a genetic predisposition and something from the environment.

A lot of the genes have been or are being defined, but lifestyle issues are very difficult to define, because it's very difficult to do that kind of clinical trial.

We do not have specific dietary recommendations for the immune system, and we do not recommend specific diets, or specific vitamins.

We know there are some vitamins that are implicated in the immune response, such as vitamins A and D.

We know that in the developing countries where vitamin deficiency is relatively common, giving vitamin A to children improves their immune response, reducing the incidence of measles, which is a major cause of death in developing countries.

That's a very specific example where supplementing with vitamin A will have a direct impact on infectious disease and immune response. That's important in the developing world, but in our country,

(continued)

unless you're on a very bizarre diet, you probably get enough vitamin A in your diet.

Vitamin D, particularly vitamin D_3, is something that immunologists are interested in because it's been shown to have an impact on immune response. But in my opinion, the average American gets plenty of vitamin D in milk and other foods, along with exposure to sunlight.

If you follow a commonsense diet that's in line with the USDA's Dietary Guidelines, and you combine that with appropriate exercise, you're doing the best job you can to keep a healthy immune system. ■

Switch In the Living Well Habits

I am a big believer in the power of small victories.

One of the keys to Living Well is taking baby steps, and opening the door to good habits, a few at a time.

Once you focus on adding the good stuff into your lifestyle, like veggies, fruits, fish, whole grains, and regular exercise, I think you'll notice something fantastic happen to your body—you may naturally and automatically have less of an appetite for junk food and processed and unhealthy foods.

Something else may happen to you, too—you'll find it a lot easier to start switching the bad stuff out, and start phasing in healthy Living Well Habits. And they all add up to make a huge difference in your life.

7 Habits of Successful Losers

There are several key habits that have fantastic promise to fulfill the crucial Living Well goal of achieving a healthy body weight.

They are based on the experience of "successful losers": the thousands of adult members of the National Weight Control Registry, all of whom have lost at least thirty pounds and kept it off for at least a year. Here are some of their biggest lessons, which are direct reflections of the Living Well Code. According to research from the Registry, many or most of the successful losers:

1. engage in high levels of physical activity, typically sixty to ninety minutes a day; favorite exercise: walking, about four miles a day;
2. eat a diet that is low in calories and moderately low in fat;
3. eat breakfast every day; favorite: cereal and fruit;
4. self-weigh regularly, at least weekly;
5. don't keep the weight off with a formal diet program, but instead adopt healthy eating patterns to enjoy for the long term;
6. watch relatively minimal TV, fewer than ten hours a week;
7. keep a food diary.

Here is a laundry list of more Living Well Habits I suggest you consider phasing into your life. Don't try them all at once, obviously!

Choose easier ones to start off with, and then add new habits as you feel comfortable.

LIVING WELL HABITS
Think Smart:

- Food is not your enemy—the right foods are a beautiful indulgence that will make you feel spectacular and live longer, healthier, and happier.
- Realize that Living Well isn't that complicated. The trouble is that we sometimes get stuck in the wrong habits, which can be corrected with a series of small tweaks.
- Don't skip meals, especially breakfast. It backfires, since you get weaker and hungrier later in the day and you wind up eating more calories.

- Don't go on a restrictive fad diet. Instead, adopt healthy eating and lifestyle habits you can live with and enjoy over the long term.
- Forget crash diets, which don't work over the long term either, and usually backfire. Don't try to lose twenty-one pounds in twenty-one days—that's an unrealistic, and possibly unhealthy, target. A healthier, more sustainable goal, for example, is to lose 10 percent of your body weight in six months. Experts also say losing a pound or two a week is a healthy weight-loss goal.
- Don't try to overhaul your whole lifestyle overnight. Allow yourself time to change.
- Don't overdeprive yourself or live in irrational fear of "bad foods." If you have a cookie or doughnut now and then, fine. Allow yourself occasional splurges, treats, and indulgences. It's all about balance—if you want, enjoy hamburgers and French fries, but as more occasional treats, not as your daily diet.
- Listen to your belly: eat until you're satisfied, not until you're totally stuffed, or you "eat everything on your plate," as Mom used to say.
- Steer clear of "comfort eating" in front of the TV or computer screen, and "emotional eating" because you're sad or bored.
- If you smoke, stop today. Don't wait for tomorrow. Cigarette smoking is the most preventable cause of premature death in the United States today. Quit right now. You can do it!
- Know your stats: go to the doctor for a thorough checkup and learn your current blood pressure, cholesterol levels, body mass index and waist circumference, fasting blood sugar level, and other key stats.
- Eat out less. When you eat out too much, you abdicate control of portions and ingredients.
- To fight stress, instead of porking out on junk food, try getting some exercise. Also experiment with natural stress-reducers like yoga, tai chi, and deep breathing. Spend your time with enthusiastic, positive, life-affirming people, and limit the time you spend with negative people.

Choose Smart:

- Think of veggies and fruits as flat-out superstars of your diet, not as bit players or costars.
- Create colorful plates where a rainbow of vegetables dazzles your eyes.
- Eat salads and soups chock-full of veggies, including leafy greens.
- When you're pressed for time, grab veggies that are quick to fix, like prewashed salad bags.
- Plan some meals around a main veggie dish, like a stir-fry.
- Include extra veggies and beans in meat loaf, stews, gravies, pasta sauces, casseroles, and lasagnas.
- Garnish plates or serving dishes with vegetable slices.
- To max up your nutrients, select a wide range of different-colored vegetables each day: greens, reds, purples, yellows, oranges.
- Have a fruit salad for dessert.
- Downsize portions of meat and poultry, and boost the vegetables, beans, and whole grains.
- Eat less processed meat like bacon, sausage, ham, and salami—and more beans, fish, and lean poultry.
- When you have meat, enjoy smaller portions and leaner cuts.
- Add more beans and less beef to your chili. Make a stir-fry with more vegetables and brown rice and less chicken. Add beans to soups, casseroles, and sauces to boost texture and flavor.
- Enjoy more whole-grain products.
- Choose low-fat and no-fat dairy products: milk, yogurts, and cheese.
- Start switching in healthier choices, and minimizing saturated and trans fats, sodium, processed foods, added sugar, and cholesterol in your diet.
- Substitute vegetables, fruits, and other low-calorie foods and beverages for foods like pizza, ice cream, doughnuts, candy, and sweetened sodas.

Shop Smart:

- Plan your shopping ahead, and write a shopping list, so you don't wander and overdo it on indulgence items in the store. You'll spend less and stay on track for healthier choices.
- Buy fewer processed foods, prepared meals, and takeaway, which are often unhealthier choices.
- In the store, spend more quality time in the fruit and veggie section than in the other departments.
- Load up your cart with more fresh produce, whole grains, and fish. Skip or breeze through the inside aisles of the market, which usually feature costly, less healthy packaged and processed foods.
- Eat before you go shopping, so you aren't tempted by high-calorie junk foods.
- Load up on frozen and canned vegetables, too, so you have them on hand anytime.
- Go to farmers' markets—they are gold mines of superfresh, seasonal produce.
- Don't be fooled by health claims on the front of food packages. Remember, "low-fat" or "nonfat" is not the same thing as "low-calorie." Low-fat foods can be high in calories.
- Shop with the Living Well Nutrition Facts Cheat Sheet on page 223 and focus on the key stats on the Nutrition Facts labels—calories, fats, sodium, cholesterol, fiber, and nutrients.
- If your supermarket offers prepared meals without full Nutrition Facts on the package, complain to the manager or e-mail the CEO that you won't buy them without this critical info.
- Shop for whole-grain rice, bread, pasta, and cereals; limit pastries, sweetened cereals, and other high-sugar foods.

Cook Smart:

- Use your microwave to "zap" veggies, fast and easy. You can nuke a delicious white or sweet potato this way, plus many other veggies. Don't worry about Internet claims that microwaving damages food. It's an urban myth. Check your microwave's veggie cooking instructions.
- Learn how to cook again! Buy a low-fat, vegetarian, Asian, or Mediterranean diet cookbook and learn new ways to enjoy your favorite foods—like stir-frying veggies.
- Instead of salt, season with herbs, spices, lemon, and other salt-free seasonings.
- Use fats and oils sparingly. Instead of cooking with butter or animal fat, cook with small amounts of extra-virgin olive oil, canola oil, safflower oil, or other healthy vegetable oils.
- Don't deep-fry foods. Instead of frying, bake, broil, roast, steam, or stew.
- Try enjoying some raw veggies in your diet.
- Steaming veggies is an especially healthy cooking method.
- Serve smaller portions of meat—remember, a standard portion is 3 ounces, about the size of a deck of cards.
- Prepare smaller portions of desserts; cut back gradually.
- Use as little water as possible when you cook veggies. If you use the cooking water for sauce or soup, you'll recapture some of the lost vitamins and minerals that leach into the water.

LIVING WELL CHECKOFF: DAY 18

I will take little tweaks and small steps and make gradual changes to switch Living Well Habits into my lifestyle.

Check Here: _____

LIVING WELL EXPERT
Patience White, M.D.

Dr. Patience White is the chief public health officer of the Arthritis Foundation.

The Arthritis Foundation is the nation's largest national non-profit health agency working on behalf of the 66 million Americans with arthritis and related diseases. Dr. White has authored numerous books and articles in such publications as the *New England Journal of Medicine and Pediatrics*, and she is also a professor of medicine and pediatrics at the George Washington University School of Medicine and Health Sciences.

Arthritis is the number-one cause of disability in America. In the worst outcome, you have to quit your job, you can't work, you can't move around, and when you do move you are in constant pain. Just imagine what it would be like if every time you moved, you hurt. What would that do to your lifestyle?

Arthritis can kill your ability to be independent. For some people—particularly baby boomers, who always want to be young and active—being dependent on others is just as bad as dying. Arthritis is also a silent partner in exacerbating many other chronic diseases, because once your arthritis keeps you from exercising, you have a very hard time doing the recommended activities you need to do to control heart disease, diabetes, and obesity.

The positive news is that if you adopt an overall healthy eating pattern, you keep your weight low, and you're physically active, you can lessen the poor outcome of your arthritis considerably.

A healthy body weight is essential in decreasing pain, improving well-being, and decreasing the progression of the most common form of

(continued)

arthritis, osteoarthritis. There is some genetic contribution to the risk for osteoarthritis, but your joint alignment, weight, physical-activity level, and history of prior injuries all play a role. And healthy weight and physical activity are central. The rate of arthritis goes up as you're heavier.

Another major type of arthritis, rheumatoid arthritis, can be controlled by drugs, but you still need to do the physical activity and stay at a healthy body weight to guard against the secondary osteoarthritis that can follow.

There is an absolute relationship here, and it's extremely important: keeping your weight in the ideal range and doing regular physical activity will decrease the progression of osteoarthritis and decrease pain and disability. The physical activity should be low-impact, like thirty minutes of walking or swimming, five to seven days a week. You can even split it up into three ten-minute blocks a day to fit into your lifestyle.

There is no diet that's going to make your arthritis go away. You'll hear all these personal testimonials: try this ginger, or ginkgo biloba, or don't eat nightshades, or eat more or less tomatoes, or get bee sting therapy. The problem is that arthritis symptoms aren't steady, they can flare up and down, and today you can feel better than you did yesterday. And some people jump to the conclusion, Oh, my, I'm much better today because yesterday I didn't eat any tomatoes.

Our advice is, eat a healthy diet, which will strengthen your bones, muscles, and joints.

All persons with arthritis, young and old, can benefit from eating a healthy, well-balanced diet. This includes a variety of foods; plenty of vegetables, fruits, and whole-grain products; and sugar, salt, and fat (especially saturated fat found in animal products) in moderation. Taking the recommended daily amounts of vitamins and minerals is also an important part of a healthful diet. A good diet promotes overall health and helps to control weight. ■

Build a Protective Environment for Your Family

was in the supermarket the other day, and I saw something that blew my mind.

There in the frozen-food section was a product called Kid Cuisine Mac and Cheese.

Hey, Kid Cuisine! Sounds like a great idea—a TV dinner designed for kids! It had an action-packed, colorful package featuring a cartoon character and nice-looking food photography. I flipped the package to check out the Nutrition Facts label and the ingredients list.

I was horrified.

This goop had over fifty ingredients listed, including, are you ready for this, carnauba wax. They use that stuff in candy corn, but they also use it to wax cars. The sodium level was 750 milligrams—which is high in sodium by adult standards! It's one thing for a consenting adult to consume this kind of food, but this is marketed expressly for our little children. How twisted is that? Is it any wonder our kids are growing up fat and sick?

Our society can be a nutrition and exercise horror movie for our families. We are increasingly prisoners inside our cars, SUVs, and BarcaLoungers, condemned to sedentary lives and overprocessed foods.

It doesn't have to be this way. I'm telling you, not one child in America will ever be able to do anything about his health and his weight unless his parents help.

We have to take charge, take back our lives, and defend our families against unhealthy habits and lifestyles. We've got to defend our home forts, seal them off from destructive forces, and build a healthy, happy home environment for our families.

It's time we turned our homes into gardens of health and delicious food, so our kids can grow into active, powerful, happy people.

Because you're a parent and role model, it's all up to you.

You are the example your kids will admire and follow.

You are responsible for what food is brought into the house—*and what food isn't.*

You should make healthy eating and physical activity a lifelong habit for your whole family. Project a positive, highly enthusiastic mind-set that tells your kids that it feels great and it is totally fun. As Crosby, Stills, Nash, and Young put it, "Teach your children well."

Show your kids that you don't skip breakfast, that veggies and fruits are a routine, tasty, no-big-deal part of your life, and that you get out and move your butt regularly. If Dad is saying, "Yuk, I never eat greens," he may be dooming his kids to a life without enjoying these magnificent gifts from God, which happen to be crucial to their health.

Healthy eating is essential to enable your child to grow, learn, think, focus, concentrate, achieve well at school and in sports, have energy, and feel happy.

Exercise with your child. Many parents don't even attempt to do that, but exercise is critical to making your children healthy. As soon as you come home from work, chase your kids out of the house for a twenty-minute power walk.

Get the whole family involved and have your own workout team, ride your bikes together, skate, challenge each other to a push-up contest. Whether it be walking or playing with your children outside in a swing at the playground, you can do it! Chasing your little toddlers around the grass for an hour is exercise.

You should break the rules. Think about it, and I mean really think—is there any reason on Earth that there should be chocolate-chip cookies, candy bars, ice cream, potato chips, junk food, or sweetened beverages in your house, except as extremely occasional items? Then don't let them in the house! Just because the rest of your block has this stuff clogging up their pantries doesn't mean you must, too. Remember, you're the leader and the gatekeeper.

You've got to defend your family!

And while you're at it, be sure to make it fun.

Tips for Living Well as a Family

- Help your children develop good healthy eating and physical activity habits at an early age by setting a good example yourself.
- Discuss highlights of this book with your children, and review the Living Well Code, the Living Well Shopping List, and the Living Well Nutrition Facts Cheat Sheet with them.
- Make your kitchen a sanctuary. Ban soda and diet soda from the house. Clear out your refrigerator and cupboards of junk food. Keep things like chips, ice cream, cookies, and pretzels out of the house except for rare occasions. Make sure you've got healthy snack options on hand at home.
- Compliment your kids when they choose healthy foods and when they get physical activity.
- Make sure everyone in the family has a healthy breakfast before leaving the house—no excuses!
- Remember, for good health, kids should ideally get at least sixty minutes of physical activity every day. All kinds of activities count, so

encourage kids to get moving by walking fast, running, dancing, jumping rope, riding bikes, skating, biking, snowboarding, swimming, playing basketball and soccer—even climbing stairs.

- Be active as a family, together. Visit the park, or throw a football or baseball. Take a family bike ride. Head out for a family walk or bike ride after dinner. Start a tradition of taking a walk after holiday meals.
- Create a rumpus room: a comfortable, safe place inside the house where kids can rock out and be active—fill it with Nerf balls, Nerf discs, Hula-Hoops and other activity toys.
- If your kids are obese or overweight, listen to what they say about their weight and their image of themselves. Empathize with them, and tell them you love and accept them no matter what their size is.
- Don't use food as a punishment or reward. An overweight kid should not feel forbidden from or deprived of food, since that could trigger food hoarding and emotional problems.
- Reassure your child that you will not put him on a diet, but that together you'll explore healthy food patterns that will be delicious and satisfying. The goal is not punishment or deprivation, but true enjoyment.
- Make fast food, prepared meals, and takeaway an occasional venture, not a way of life.
- Put stealth veggies in spaghetti sauce, vegetable stir-fries, bean burritos, and soups—not to be sneaky, but as a no-big-deal way of making things taste better and enjoying more vegetables.
- Turn your kids on to healthy fruit and veggie smoothies.
- Involve your kids in grocery shopping, meal planning, and meal preparation.
- In the supermarket, ask children to pick new vegetables, fruits, and whole grains to try.
- Let children decide on the dinner vegetables or what goes into salads.
- If they're old enough, children can help clean, peel, and cut up vegetables.

- Invite the kids to help you cook. Give them a manageable task, like scrambling the eggs or rinsing the strawberries. Younger kids can tear lettuce for a salad or drop a dollop of yogurt on top of fruit.
- Start a vegetable garden so your children can pick and eat the vegetables they grow.
- Take your kids to the farmers' market and ask the vendors to explain where some of the foods come from. Visit a working farm and show your kids how their food is grown.
- Serve cut-up vegetables as part of an afternoon snack.
- Eat your meals together as a family, at the dinner table. Switch off the TV and computers. Eat slowly, and enjoy the food, the conversation, and the laughter.
- When it comes to healthy living, provide structure; set rules and boundaries for your kids to follow.
- Try the power of ten to fifteen. That's the average number of times a child needs to try a new food before liking it, according to experts.
- Don't get into bargaining games. If you say, "Eat your vegetable, and then you can have dessert," you're just getting into a food power struggle that you can't win over the long term.
- Get the whole family involved in healthy eating and regular physical activity. Don't single out one child, even if the others aren't overweight. You all need to develop good habits.
- Encourage your child to take part in activities that involve moving, not sitting. Set limits on how much time they spend watching TV, playing video games, and surfing the Internet.
- If you drive your kids to school, try walking with them sometimes instead.
- If your kids' school doesn't have regular physical education classes and a strong healthy eating program featuring delicious healthy food, call the principal and ask why. Work with your school to make it better. Organize with other parents and change things for the better.

LIVING WELL CHECKOFF: DAY 19

As the leader and role model, I will start building a protective home environment for my family, get them to live an active lifestyle, and transform my kitchen into a garden of health, beauty, and delicious flavors for my children to enjoy.

Check Here: _____

LIVING WELL EXPERT
David S. Ludwig, M.D., Ph.D.

Dr. David S. Ludwig is director of the Optimal Weight for Life (OWL) Program at Children's Hospital Boston and associate professor of pediatrics at Harvard Medical School.

He is an authority on childhood obesity, and is the author of Ending the Food Fight: Guide Your Child to a Healthy Weight in a Fast Food/Fake Food World.

Dr. Ludwig's OWL Clinic has treated five thousand families over the past twelve years, many of them from lower-income or minority communities. He has published seventy-five articles in medical or scientific journals, including the *Journal of the American Medical Association (JAMA)*, the *New England Journal of Medicine*, and the *Lancet*.

Dr. Ludwig makes a huge point: we have to build protective home environments for ourselves and our children, and get the junk out of our homes.

When I started down this path of healthy eating, I went to my kitchen and I cleaned all the crap out. I got rid of all the processed, high-fat, and high-sodium foods, the white bread, everything unhealthy I thought I might get up at two o'clock in the morning and pork out on. Instead of raiding the refrigerator for junk food in the middle of the night, I'll reach for a cold blended vegetable-and-fruit drink. I'm serious. I stock my refrigerator with them five or six at a time!

We live in a toxic environment.

The irony is that on the one hand, we're told that childhood obesity is a top public health emergency that, unaddressed, will have a devastating impact on life expectancy and national health-care costs. But on the other hand, families with overweight children are being undermined at every step, with incessant junk-food advertising aimed at young children, a school lunch program often resembling a fast-food restaurant, and cutbacks or elimination of physical education programs.

When it comes to junk-food advertising, the issue is clearly not one of First Amendment rights, as has been established by the courts with respect to tobacco. The food industry should not have a blank check to advertise unhealthful products to our children.

These products have the worst possible nutritional quality, and are loaded with hydrogenated (trans) fats, concentrated sugars, highly refined starches, and a host of artificial additives. They're extremely high in calorie density and low in quality, with few if any vitamins, minerals, and antioxidants. Study after study has clearly demonstrated that this eating pattern has a major impact on risk for obesity, diabetes, heart disease, and even cancer.

We all need to work together to make our environment a healthier place to live. It's everybody's responsibility. But until the politicians in Washington and the food industry place public health before short-term financial considerations, it's up to parents to protect their children from this toxic environment.

The most important parenting practice, in my opinion, is protecting the home environment.

(continued)

Protecting the home environment means making healthful eating and physical activity easy and convenient, and unhealthful habits much less so.

Stock your home with an abundance of fresh vegetables and fruits, beans, seeds, nuts and nut butters, whole grains, and healthy proteins. Put fresh fruit in a bowl at the front of the refrigerator, place a bowl of nuts and dried fruit on a counter. Chop up carrots, celery, broccoli, cauliflower, and bell peppers, and arrange them on a plate next to some really tasty dips.

You don't have to eliminate sweet treats entirely. Go out for ice cream once in a while and make it a celebration, but don't keep it in the house. Remember, you can either say no to the carton of ice cream once, when your kids ask you for it in the supermarket, or you can try to say no every night when the kids nag you for it if it's sitting in the freezer.

Turn off the TV (and get it out of the bedrooms and kitchen). Instead, create a play station in the corner of the living room with games, toys, and music that support physical activity.

I find it ironic that many people think healthy eating and an active lifestyle are inconvenient. The alternatives are so much more inconvenient.

An obese adolescent with type 2 diabetes may need to check blood sugars many times a day and inject insulin. Without adequate management, diabetes can cause heart attack, stroke, kidney failure, blindness, and other very "inconvenient" complications.

The beauty of protecting the home environment is that everyone benefits: the overweight child loses weight and reduces risk for diabetes, a lean sibling avoids a future weight problem, and parents' blood pressure and cholesterol improve.

Try it—it's easier than you think! ■

Live Well on the Run

run around the United States a lot on business trips, and I come face-to-face with the most delicious, belly-busting food our country has to offer.

I just got back from a trip down South, where you'll find some of the nicest people and most gigantic food portions in the world.

Mmmmmm . . . Southern cookin'. Grandma's buttermilk biscuits in the oven. Baby back ribs on the barbecue. Deep-fried chicken slathered with gravy. Carrots cooked with butter and brown sugar. Sweet potato pie. This stuff is so delicious and the plates are so enormous that if I lived there, I wonder if I'd be the size of a small house.

Let me ask you something: how in the heck are we supposed to eat healthy when we're faced with all these tempting choices? How are we supposed to eat healthy when we've got to get the kids off to school, drive an hour to the office, and manage our jobs and our families in an overstressed, 24/7 BlackBerry world? We've barely got time to sleep!

We need to Live Well when we're on the run: when we eat breakfast, when we're grabbing snacks, traveling, eating out, and making fast meals.

Living Well on the run starts with breakfast. Breakfast is where it all begins. You can't run out the door without a good basic breakfast.

When you wake up, your body has been on a twelve-hour fast and it craves good energy in the form of healthy food. "A healthy breakfast has been shown to help with energy, weight, mood and the ability to think," notes Dr. Ken Fujioka, the director of nutrition and metabolic research at Scripps Clinic in San Diego.

Be good to yourself. You simply cannot skip breakfast. Skipping breakfast makes you weak, and over time it may very well make you fat, because you overcompensate by overeating later in the day.

We've got to get breakfast every morning—but we should feel free to break the rules.

I've had to fight a battle with myself to get out of the straitjacket conventions of breakfast.

Let me tell you: I grew up on eggs, bacon, sausage, and potatoes. Baby, that was it! If you didn't have that, it wasn't breakfast. Breakfast became my comfort food, my big meal and dessert of the day. At the Naval Academy, I'd have eggs, bacon, and waffles with ice cream for breakfast! How sick is that? Five years ago it would not have been abnormal for my son and me to go to the Olympic Diner in New York City and order a waffle with some ice cream and syrup, and an omelet filled with sausage, bacon, and cheese!

We've got to get out of the habit of being forced to eat what we've been advertised is breakfast food. As a society we've somehow decided that we have to have sausage, ham, greasy fried potatoes, and jumbo bagels with cream cheese for breakfast. We've declared them to be breakfast foods.

These are not healthy breakfasts. Over time, they are a first-class ticket to a potbelly, heart disease, or worse. It's like chugalugging artery-clogging saturated fat, cholesterol, and tons of sugar. I don't think human beings were evolved to go to IHOP and have a mountain of pancakes soaked in butter and syrup every morning.

We're actually genetically programmed to have simple, fresh, whole foods in the morning. Thousands of years ago, we had a bunch of fruit left over from the day before when we went out hunting, and that was our breakfast.

We should declare war on bad breakfasts.

I believe you should eat whatever you want in the morning as long as it's healthy. I have egg whites three days a week; I have granola with nut milk once or twice a week. Sometimes it's vegetable or miso soup. I mix my breakfasts up. I don't want the same thing every day.

When I shifted over to healthy, light breakfasts, I started feeling great instead of sluggish.

Personally, I like eggs. I don't think eggs are bad for you if you eat them in moderation, and you focus on egg whites like I do. Some mornings, whitefish becomes my bacon or sausage—sautéed or poached in olive oil with capers. You heard me: fish for breakfast. Try it. It's great! If you like fish at six at night, why wouldn't it taste good at seven thirty a.m.?

I usually have one of my blended fruit-and-vegetable drinks in the morning, too. You might be thinking, *Montel, are you serious? I'm not going to drink a Green Drink every morning after I get out of bed!* OK, then don't! Have your fruit and oatmeal, or berries and granola, or egg white on whole-grain toast.

Living Well Breakfast Tips

- Plain, unsweetened, whole-grain oatmeal is a breakfast superstar. Filling and easy to fix, it boasts fiber and other nutrients. Sweeten it up with fresh berries and fruit, and add in some low-fat or fat-free yogurt if you like. Also try oatmeal with nuts, low-fat or fat-free milk, or a soy-based beverage, with cottage cheese on the side.
- Try some low-fat yogurt sprinkled with low-fat granola.
- Have a fruit-and-vegetable smoothie.
- If you're used to having breakfast meat like sausage or bacon every morning, why not go from once a day to every third day, and try an option like turkey sausage links?

- Have some whole-grain toast with a thin spread of nut butter or peanut butter.
- Go for a high-fiber, low-sugar, whole-grain cold cereal with a minimum of 8 grams of fiber per serving.
- If you're feeling extremely adventurous, break the rules completely and have a 100 percent vegetable-and-whole-grain-based breakfast, like a microwaved sweet potato, some microwaved low-sodium canned beans, and a ninety-second microwaveable brown rice pouch. I know it sounds totally insane, but try it and see how great you feel at midmorning.
- Be the first person in the history of your town to have healthy, omega-3-packed Alaskan salmon right out of the can with your breakfast instead of greasy bacon. It's such a shocking and brilliant idea you may make page one of the local paper.
- Try an instant healthy "caveman breakfast" of three grab-and-go fruits: one banana, one apple, and one peach.

When you're away from home, it's really hard to eat healthy. It does require a shift in your thinking, in some of your basic assumptions and your behavior. But I tell you, the payoff is really worth it.

When I'm on the road I do whatever I can to eat healthy. I load up on salads, I take healthy granola bars along with me in my briefcase, and I even pack bottles of my Green Drinks into flexible cooler bags with ice packs and check it in at the airport gate.

Living Well Eating-Out Tips

- When you eat out, choose restaurants that offer nutritional info and healthier options.
- If a chain restaurant refuses to give you calorie and other nutritional info, get up and leave. It's time we all started voting with our feet and requiring all restaurant chains to treat our health with respect.

- Ask questions about the menu. If you like, try an experiment that often works for me (I'm not sure if it's because I'm a celebrity or because the waiters are so nice!): ask if it's possible for the restaurant to make you a big salad with the freshest different veggies they have on hand, perhaps garnished with some chicken, fish, or beans.
- Instead of eating out at the office, pack your own lunch a few times a week, like a sandwich made with whole-grain bread or wrap, fish or chicken, and packed with lots of extra veggies.
- Use the principles of the Living Well Code to guide your ordering: go for more veggies, fruits, and whole grains; ask for fish, beans, or leaner cuts of poultry and meat; watch calories and try to minimize saturated fat, sodium, and cholesterol.
- Skip the salt shaker. Flavor your food with lemon, herbs, pepper, or other nonsalt options.
- Ask for your meal to be prepared without salt. Don't be embarrassed to ask—you're spending your good, hard-earned money on that food!
- In the coffee shop, keep a close eye on calories: a Starbucks venti Java Chip Frappuccino has 650 calories, which can completely blow your day's calorie balance.
- In restaurants, don't supersize; downsize instead. Lots of restaurants serve portions that are double or triple the proper healthy size. Split your plate with your partner or ask for a doggie bag.
- Skip the 1,000-calorie desserts like cheesecake or a fudge brownie sundae.
- To minimize calories and fat, ask for foods that are steamed, grilled, broiled, or lightly sautéed or stir-fried—rather than foods that are deep-fried or "crispy."
- Skip the soda. Just because the average American drinks fifty-six gallons of soda a year(!), there's no reason you should. As Dr. Meir Stampfer of the Harvard School of Public Health once put it, "We ought to think of soft drinks as a treat, like ice cream, not as a staple."

• Go for plain iced water from the tap, unsweetened iced tea with lemon, lightly flavored seltzer, nonfat milk, or sparkling water.

When you're working hard and pressed for time, it's easy to fall into an unhealthy snack rut of candy bars, potato chips, salty snacks, and alleged "energy bars" with too much saturated fat and calories.

Here are some ideas for Living Well while you snack.

Living Well Snack Tips

• Don't be afraid to snack between meals, but make them healthy. Vegetables and fruits are the earth's original masterpiece snack foods. Grab 'em and go.
• Instead of a gooey pastry, snack on a fruit cup, a bunch of grapes, or an orange.
• Keep a bowl of washed, chopped-up veggies in your refrigerator for fast mouthfuls: baby carrots, celery sticks, cooked sweet potato chunks, chopped greens.
• Instead of a candy bar or bag of cookies, fire up a fast smoothie.
• Just say no to vending machines; most of the stuff inside is large portions of pretty useless stuff—potato chips, candy, cookies. Instead, make your own little Baggies of trail mix for the week ahead and pack them in your Briefcase or purse for fast, indulgent energy snacks. Make your own trail mix from raisins, walnuts, peanuts, almonds, sunflower seeds, dried apricots or cranberries, and other dried fruits, unsalted nuts, and seeds. Watch the portion sizes, as the calories in nuts can add up if you overdo it.
• Keep packages of potato chips, nacho chips, candy, cookies, doughnuts, and ice cream out of your house except for special occasions. Better yet, skip them altogether. If it's there, let's face it, you're going to eat it.

- Look for a healthy snack you can really enjoy and stick with, like a lower-calorie granola or fruit bar, for example.
- Never eat snacks right out of a big bag. You won't know when to stop, and before you know it you'll have eaten far more than you should have.
- With so-called energy bars, check the Nutrition Facts label and watch out for items with too much saturated fat, sodium, or sugar.
- Enjoy snacking on some nonfat cheese and whole-grain bread or crackers.

Why do we buy prepackaged convenience foods?

To save time, right?

Guess what—convenience foods may save some shopping time, but at home they may not save us much time at all.

According to a surprising study by UCLA researchers published in the July 2007 issue of the *British Medical Journal*, working families rely heavily on "convenience" foods for dinner, but save little time. The study examined the behavior of thirty-two middle-class families with working parents. The researcher Dr. Margaret Beck reported, "People don't spend any less time overall on dinner when they use so-called convenience foods. . . . Families seem to spend a certain amount of time cooking regardless."

How can this be? Well, paradoxically, people who used prepackaged convenience foods wound up making more elaborate meals with more different dishes, while the home cooks who made dinner from scratch made simpler dinners like one-pot dishes or healthy sandwiches. And you're probably paying two penalties for the prepackaged stuff: it's both more expensive and less healthy, with more preservatives, sodium, and saturated fat.

"The best piece of advice I give for eating healthy is to plan," commented the New Orleans physician Timothy Harlan in the *Wall Street*

Journal. "Get the ingredients in your house that will help you build something very simple." Dr. Beck of UCLA agreed. "People should give themselves a break. It's OK to put a simple meal on the table."

Simple meals. Whole foods, not processed foods, are more deeply filling. Less is more. Easy is better.

This I like!

LIVING WELL CHECKOFF: DAY 20

Starting today, I'll start applying the principles of the Living Well Code to my snacking, breakfasts, and eating on the run and eating out.

Check Here: _____

Take the Living Well Pledge

I met a wonderful young lady on my show by the name of Evelyn.

She was struggling with her weight, and she was worried about her physical appearance.

Worst of all, she was worried that she was setting a bad example for her young daughter, who already weighed 140 pounds and had a hip problem. She was just a girl.

"Both my parents are diabetic," Evelyn told me, "and they're both overweight. Diabetes runs in my family, I'm asthmatic, and my oldest daughter gets teased at school all the time for being overweight. When she walks, they yell, '*Earthquake!*'"

The teasing got so bad that this girl would come home from school crying.

I looked into Evelyn's eyes and could tell how worried she was that somehow, through her own behavior and lifestyle, she was passing a terrible health problem down to her beloved daughter.

I told Evelyn that now was the time she had to *get busy*. Because her daughter's life was literally at stake.

I believe that problems are a normal, natural product of life. Problems exist for us to grapple with, study, and analyze—and then run over. Problems make us stronger.

I believe in solutions—long-term solutions. Early in the history of *The Montel Williams Show*, we became the first TV talk show to offer a full-scale counseling program for our guests with problems.

It started in 1993 with a young woman who cut herself—she was a self-mutilator—and she was anorexic and bulimic. She came to me and said, "Montel, please help me."

I told her that she was not leaving until we found out how we could help her. That day we found a hospital, and we put her in it. It was a full-residential treatment program, and we took care of it. I'm not like some other TV hosts who say they will give you some help, which turns out to be a half hour in the greenroom after the show.

I have a full-time psychologist on my staff, and *The Montel Williams Show* is the only show of its kind to have one. Our show's After-Care Program has arranged for guests to attend psychological counseling sessions, weight-loss and eating-disorder programs, and drug rehabilitation centers after they appear on the show. We've put people through full residential-treatment programs that beat heroin and other drug addiction. We've sent people to counseling for six and seven months.

When I met Evelyn, I believed that just like you and me, she was totally capable of changing her physical destiny and her health, if she had the right information, the right help, and the right motivation. We brought Evelyn into our After-Care Program and introduced her to expert advice on healthy eating and healthy living.

A few months later, she came back on the show to show me how she was doing.

Well, let me tell you, I was overjoyed.

Evelyn looked fantastic, and she said she felt great, too. She literally glowed with positive energy. Here's what she said:

> Since the show, I have been doing much, much better.
>
> I lost twenty pounds. My self-esteem is much better. I don't get as depressed as before. I have more energy.
>
> I enjoy doing a lot of things that I didn't do before, like going out and going to the park with my daughter. And after work, I work out. I

try to work out three times a week for an hour. I try to get the best cardio I can. I try to do a lot of weights.

I stick to my three meals a day and two snacks in between. I eat a lot of salad, a lot of vegetables, which I wouldn't do before.

I spend more time with my kids. I feel more alive. It's important because, as you know, my parents are sick and my daughter is overweight. And it's helped me immensely to see that I, at least, could help my daughter's weight by setting an example.

Being on the show really did change my life. And because of Montel, I made it this far.

Do you remember the Quance family I told you about in chapter two? The entire family was overweight and extremely concerned about their health and the amount of junk food they were eating.

After we taped that show, the Quance family left the studio with a new healthy attitude about their lifestyle. But I wanted to check in to see if it continued after they left. So a few months later, we sent our cameras back into their house.

What we found was absolutely beautiful. We found a family transforming their lives for the better.

"Being on the show, I learned a lot of different stuff," reported Dale, the chocolate-and-soda-pop-loving dad who had been overweight for years. Now he reported, "I've lost about fourteen pounds by watching what I eat, and not gorging myself and finishing everything on my plate." He added, "We try to eat more fruits and vegetables, and healthy meat, instead of always going out to eat and eating junk food."

Dale's wife, Melissa, was glowing with pride over her family's achievement-in-progress: "I have lost twelve pounds since the show. It makes me feel great. That makes me want to lose more. So now I really want to discipline myself even more. It's worth it to live a longer, healthier life, and to see the kids be a lot healthier. And they look a lot healthier—they won't get so picked on about being overweight."

Their daughter Brittany summed it up beautifully: "Since I lost the weight, I'm less tired. I've got a lot more energy. Each pound I lose, I gain a little bit more confidence."

How great is that?

Living Well really works!

If there's one thing I want you to take away from this book, it's that you are the only person who owns the definition of who you are physically.

You can take your physical fate into your own hands and transform it for the better.

It's up to you, not your doctors, to take control of your health.

I get up every single day and work out as hard as I can. Every day is a struggle. And I'm in it to win it. Period.

I work out almost every day, just so I can fake you out. I've been as public as I can possibly be about the fact that I have MS, but I just don't want you to see me limp. So I work as hard as I can, and I eat as healthy as I can. Because Living Well makes me feel healthy and fantastic.

Sometimes the obstacles we face in life can seem like the biggest mountaintop. They can seem too huge to ever overcome. But if you have faith in yourself, and you get some knowledge and education, you can beat them.

Let me tell you something: once you make the decision to truly start Living Well, there's nothing your family can't do, there's nothing at work you can't do, there's nothing at school you can't do, and there's nothing in your life you can't change.

That's why I'm always saying, "Mountain, get out of my way."

I will not take no for an answer!

When you're born, you cry and the world rejoices.

The key is to live your life so that when you die, the world cries and you can rejoice.

I want to rejoice the whole way.

We dedicate ourselves to our jobs, and we dedicate ourselves to other people—why can't we dedicate ourselves to ourselves? To making our life the best it can be?

I'm going to be fifty-two years old this year. I don't regret any day of those years, including the day that I was diagnosed with a major illness, because that has made me learn more about myself and human nature than I would have learned in my entire life. I wouldn't trade it for a thing.

What gives me peace is the knowledge that whatever happens, I will be the person that defines who I am, period.

I have one last exercise for you.

Read the Living Well Pledge, check off each point, and place a copy in your family scrapbook or photo album, or on the center of the refrigerator door.

TAKE THE LIVING WELL PLEDGE

What I Now Know

• I know that Living Well can reduce my risk for a host of killer diseases. _____

• I know that Living Well can transform my life, extend my lifespan, and help me feel spectacular. _____

• I know that crash diets and fad diets don't work, nor does skipping meals, cutting out food groups, or torturing myself.

_____

• I know that calories count for health and for healthy weight.

_____

(continued)

- I know that Living Well physically means healthy eating and regular physical activity, not a magic pill. _____

- I know that Living Well is not a quick fix—it is a lifetime pursuit. _____

- I know that food is not my enemy—it is a source of joy, health, and delicious physical pleasure. _____

- I know that it is up to me to take charge of my own health and my family's health. _____

What I Will Now Do

- I will base my diet on a rich variety of many vegetables and fruits. _____

- I will eat whole grains as a source of healthy energy and good carbohydrates. _____

- I will include in my diet foods like fish, beans, and nuts.

  _____

- I will pay attention to nutrition labels. _____

- I will be mindful of my calories in and calories out to work toward a healthy body weight. _____

- I will work toward the goal of enjoying regular physical activity: at least thirty to sixty minutes of moderate exercise on most days of the week. _____

- I will work with a doctor and/or dietitian on my goals.
  _____

- I will not skip meals, especially breakfast. _____

- I will say no to diet concepts that are not based on healthy eating. _____

- I will say no to diet concepts that are not based on real evidence from real experts. _____

- I will look for health and nutrition information based on good evidence, not on anecdotes only. _____

- I will allow myself indulgences and treats. _____

- I will begin switching in healthier choices, and switching out saturated and trans fats, sodium, processed foods, added sugars, and cholesterol from my diet. _____

- I will involve my family in Living Well. _____

- I will build a protective home environment for my family that encourages Living Well. _____

- I will start to Live Well for Life by adopting healthy lifetime attitudes. _____

Congratulations—you've made it to Day 21.

You've already surpassed by four days the time frame that experts say it takes to change a habit. If you can do something for seventeen days or more, it's a habit.

So now that you're on the other side, recognize what you've already been able to accomplish, and use this as your launch pad for the next cycle of twenty-one days, and the next cycle, and the next.

For the last twenty-one days you gave yourself a gift—the gift of starting to Live Well. Now imagine what a wonderful gift it would be to give to your family, too—to your spouse, kids, your mom and dad. How beautiful would it be to spend many more golden, healthy days enjoying life with them?

Do you remember back on Day 1 when I asked you to take some photos of yourself and file them away? Now dig them out. How do you feel today? How do you look today? Are you ready to commit to really Live Well for life?

If you're like me, on some days you'll find that Living Well is a real challenge.

But there will be other days when you'll do it perfectly—and it will be much easier than you think. I know that you're going to feel better than you felt before you started, and that's the thing that will motivate you to keep going and keep succeeding.

Keep taking small steps, making small improvements, and savoring small victories.

If you stick with this, the rewards are incalculably huge—living longer, fighting off diseases, staying out of the hospital, and enjoying a rich, independent, action-packed life, which all add up to a much more beautiful way to live.

You now have the power to transform your life, supercharge your health, and feel spectacular.

The power is in your hands.

It's time to unleash the power, right now!

LIVING WELL WEEKLY PLANNER FOOD AND ACTIVITY DIARY

Notes:

	MON	TUE	WED	THU	FRI	SAT	SUN
BREAKFAST							
LUNCH							
DINNER							
ALL OTHER: *Snacks, Lattes, Candy, Liquid Candy (Sugared Beverages), Office Munchies, etc.*							
PHYSICAL ACTIVITY TYPE:							
HOW MANY MINUTES:							

MY SPECIFIC PLANS TO LIVE WELL THIS WEEK:

The kinds of foods I'll enjoy:

The physical activities I'll enjoy:

The behaviors I'll make better:

The attitudes I'll make better:

Ways I'll help my family live well:

More Living Well
Recipes

Here are more of my favorite recipes for the Living Well lifestyle.

They are culinary celebrations of the themes of vegetables, fruits, whole grains, and lean, healthy protein. They are also nutritious, filling, and in my opinion completely indulgent!

Many of the recipes in this book were developed with my executive chef, Mike Schurr, and several others were created by the nutritional experts at the American Institute for Cancer Research.

I hope you'll try these recipes as delicious additions to your family's menu, and I also hope they'll serve as inspirations for you to explore your own path to healthy, delicious eating.

Bon appetit!

SOME TIPS

When following the recipes in this book:
- Read first, from start to finish.
- Ingredients are listed in the order they will be used.
- Unless otherwise instructed, assume all produce is washed thoroughly and dried first.
- Any canned or frozen ingredients should contain no added salt or sugar.

WASH ALL FRUITS AND VEGETABLES WELL: Swish greens in a large bowl of cold water. Grit will settle at the bottom of the bowl. Lift out the greens, drain bowl, and repeat until no grit remains.

TRY NEW SALAD GREENS: Make a salad with greens you know you like. Then, add one unfamiliar green to the mix at a time so you can grow accustomed to new flavors.

PREPARING RAW CORN: Remove the silk by brushing downward on the cob using a paper towel. To remove kernels from cob, over a large bowl, holding shucked corn by the stem, slice from stem to tip using a sharp knife.

LOADING THE VITA-MIX OR OTHER BLENDER: To avoid jams, load liquids and soft ingredients first and start at a low speed. Then, gradually increase speed to desired level.

RAW FOODS: Soaking time can be decreased by using hot water.

HERBS: Use dried herbs in the beginning stages of cooking, allowing them ample time to reconstitute and redevelop their original flavor. Add fresh herbs at the end of cooking to help retain their flavor and freshness.

HAVE FUN AND EXPERIMENT: The process of preparing food for yourself and your loved ones will bring added health and joy. Also, try learning how to grow some of your own vegetables!

The "Big Mike" Garden Vegetable Burger with Roasted Sweet Potato Fries

*This burger looks and tastes like the real thing—only it's better for you.
It's packed with greens and proteins and topped with a "special sauce,"
much like the one featured at everybody's favorite fast-food joint. This
burger can be ready in a jiffy when pan-fried, but for a healthier version,
try it baked (just be sure to preheat the oven to 350°F before prepping the
patties). Ground flaxseeds bind the patties together and add protein, fiber,
and superhealthy omega-3s. I use a coffee/spice grinder to grind whole
flaxseeds down to a fine powder.*

SERVES 4.

GARDEN VEGETABLE PATTIES

Ingredients

12 ounces portobello mushrooms (approx. 8 med. mushrooms), quartered

1 cup frozen, shelled edamame, thawed

20 grape tomatoes

1 tablespoon parsley, coarsely chopped

1 cup sweet onion, coarsely chopped

¼ teaspoon salt

2 teaspoons ground pepper

1 cup ground golden flaxseeds or flax meal

Procedure

In a food processor, combine mushrooms, edamame, tomatoes, parsley, onion, salt, and pepper. Pulse until a ground-beef-like consistency is achieved. Transfer mixture to a medium-sized mixing bowl. Mix in ground flax and stir until well absorbed. Using your bare hands, form the mixture into four equal-sized patties. Patties may be fried in a small amount of extra-virgin olive oil over medium-high heat, flipping once, until both sides are golden brown *or* baked on a cookie sheet lined with greased parchment paper for 45–60 minutes at 350 degrees.

"SPECIAL SAUCE"

Ingredients

 ½ block firm tofu (7 ounces), halved

 3 ounces tomato paste

 1 cherry pepper, seeded and quartered

 1 clove garlic, chopped

 2 tablespoons apple cider vinegar

 2 tablespoons extra-virgin olive oil

 ¼ teaspoon salt

 1 teaspoon blackstrap molasses

 1 teaspoon brown mustard

 ¼ teaspoon low-sodium soy sauce

 ½ teaspoon raw honey or agave nectar

 juice of 2 medium lemons

Procedure

 In a food processor, combine all ingredients and process 2–3 minutes until smooth.

THE BIG MIKE

Ingredients

 8 slices low-sodium whole-grain bread

 Special Sauce

 24 ¼-inch-thick slices of low-sodium pickle

 8 leaves romaine or Boston lettuce

 1 sweet onion, sliced into ⅛-inch rounds

 4 Garden Vegetable Patties

Procedure

Align 4 pieces of bread side by side and spread a thin layer of Special Sauce and 3 pickle slices onto each. Lay down a piece of lettuce and then a slice of onion. Add a Garden Vegetable Patty on top of each onion slice. Smear one side of the remaining bread with Special Sauce. Affix bread, sauce side down, flip, and serve with a side of Roasted Sweet Potato Fries (see below).

ROASTED SWEET POTATO FRIES

Ingredients

    1 pound sweet potatoes, peeled and cut lengthwise into $\frac{1}{2}$-inch
        slices
    2 tablespoons extra-virgin olive oil
    $\frac{1}{4}$ teaspoon salt

Procedure

Preheat oven to 425°F. In a large mixing bowl, toss together sliced sweet potatoes and olive oil. Transfer to a lightly oiled cookie sheet, spread evenly, and roast, turning once, 35–40 minutes, or until fries are golden brown. Remove from oven and immediately sprinkle with salt to taste. Let cool 1 minute, then serve with a side of Special Sauce.

Raw Coriander Carrot Soup with Avocado and Fresh Herbs

When you pack in the veggies, and you hold off on the extraneous sodium, soups can be a highly nutritious, filling, and enjoyable part of your daily food life.

Here's one of my favorite soup dishes. It's so action-packed and satisfying that it can serve as a complete meal.

Carrot and coriander is a delicious pairing. With the addition of creamy avocado and the zest of fresh herbs, this quick and easy soup tastes like it takes hours to make.

Avocados are great; they have a substantial, full-bodied taste and are fine sources of heart-healthy monounsaturated fats. Avocados give me a burst of energy and help me feel nice and full. It's just a wonderful-feeling vegetable.

SERVES 3–4.

Ingredients

> 2 cups fresh carrot juice (the amount of carrots needed in this recipe will depend on your juicer's yield), carrot pulp reserved for thickening
>
> 2 avocados, peel and pit removed, cut into chunks
>
> 1/2 teaspoon salt
>
> 1/4 cup fresh parsley, stemmed
>
> 1 teaspoon coriander, ground
>
> 2 teaspoons extra-virgin olive oil
>
> 1 tablespoon cilantro, finely chopped

Procedure

In a Vita-Mix, blend carrot juice, 1 avocado, salt, parsley, and coriander until smooth. If added thickness is desired, blend in carrot pulp as necessary.

Serve chilled in soup bowls and garnish with a swirl of olive oil, a few chunks of avocado, and a sprinkle of fresh cilantro.

15-Minute Turkey Tacos

Everybody thinks it takes a long time to fix a healthy meal. But guess what. You can whip up this embarrassingly easy, healthy taco recipe from my friend and Living Well Coach Chris Freytag in fifteen minutes.

Try doing it with your kids, and give them a job to do, like chopping up the lettuce and tomatoes.

I have three words for you: basic, fast, and easy!

SERVES 2–4.

Ingredients

1 pound lean ground turkey

1 packet taco seasoning (I buy the organic kind—no weird chemicals or extra sodium)

2 cups low-fat cheddar cheese, shredded

lettuce, chopped

tomatoes, chopped

soft-shell or hard-shell tacos (I buy only the brands without partially hydrogenated oils—you have to read the label!)

salsa or taco sauce

Procedure

Brown the turkey in a nonstick skillet over medium heat. Add the seasoning according to the packet. Build your tacos—shell, turkey, cheese, lettuce, tomato, and sauce or salsa. *Yum!*

Montel's Superpower Breakfast: Raw Cinnamon Spice Cereal with Vanilla Cashew Milk

Spoon out a bowlful of raw cereal, pour on some vanilla cashew milk, top it off with a few slices of ripe banana and fresh strawberries—you've got yourself one bangin' breakfast.

SERVES 6–8.

VANILLA CASHEW MILK

Ingredients

- 1 cup raw cashews
- 3 cups water
- ½ vanilla bean or 1 teaspoon alcohol-free vanilla extract
- ⅛ teaspoon salt
- 1 tablespoon agave nectar to taste

Procedure

In a Vita-Mix, add cashews, water, vanilla, salt, and agave to taste. Blend 1 minute at high speed. (If smoother milk is desired, strain through a fine mesh strainer.) Store in a 1-quart container in the refrigerator. Keeps for 2–3 days.

RAW CINNAMON SPICE GRANOLA CEREAL

Ingredients

- 1 cup raw pumpkin seeds
- ½ cup raw sunflower seeds
- 1 cup dried pears (approx. 6 pieces) or dried apple
- 1 cup raisins
- 1 teaspoon ground cinnamon
- ¼ teaspoon salt

Procedure

In a food processor, combine all ingredients and pulse until well combined. Process for 20–30 seconds until ingredients are a similar small size.

Breakfast Burritos

This and the next three recipes are from the American Institute for Cancer Research (AICR). The AICR has a passion for tweaking our daily diet so it's tasty and really good for us, like these rocking breakfast burritos.

SERVES 4.

Ingredients

2 large eggs

4 egg whites

2 teaspoons olive oil

1 medium tomato, seeded and chopped

¼ cup green pepper, diced

¼ cup red pepper, diced

¼ cup yellow squash, diced

¼ cup green onion, chopped

salt and freshly ground black pepper, to taste

cayenne pepper, to taste (optional)

4 tablespoons soy bacon bits (or to taste)

4 flour tortillas, preferably whole wheat, room temperature or warmed

Procedure

In a medium bowl, beat eggs with egg whites. Set aside. Heat olive oil in a nonstick skillet over medium heat. When oil is hot, add tomato, peppers, squash, and onion. Cook 3 minutes, stirring constantly. Add eggs and scramble with a fork or spoon. Add salt, pepper, and cayenne, if using. When eggs are cooked, stir in soy bacon bits. Divide eggs evenly onto tortillas. Roll up tightly, burrito style, and serve immediately.

Breakfast Fruit Wrap

SERVES 1.

Ingredients

 1 tortilla, preferably whole wheat

 2 teaspoons "fruit only" strawberry preserves

 2 tablespoons reduced-fat ricotta cheese

 $\frac{1}{3}$–$\frac{1}{2}$ cup fresh strawberries, sliced

 2 tablespoons almonds, sliced and toasted

Procedure

On a surface, spread preserves on tortilla. Top with ricotta cheese. Carefully top with sliced fruit. Sprinkle with sliced almonds. Starting from one end, roll tightly. Wrap in foil for neater eating. Variation: spread tortilla with apricot preserves and use sliced fresh or canned well-drained peaches.

Broccoli, Cherry Tomato, and Watercress Salad

I'm a broccoli-resistant guy. I just can't help it. One of my New Year's resolutions this year is to work some broccoli into my life, which I've never been able to do. This recipe just may do the trick.

SERVES 4.

Ingredients

 2 cups broccoli florets

 1 tablespoon red wine vinegar

 1 tablespoon olive oil

 $\frac{1}{2}$ teaspoon minced garlic

 salt and freshly ground black pepper to taste

 2 cups cherry tomatoes, stems removed and cut in half

 1 bunch watercress, long stems trimmed, coarsely chopped

Procedure

In a vegetable steamer set over boiling water, steam broccoli, covered, until tender, about 4 minutes. Rinse with cold water; drain well. In a large bowl, whisk vinegar, olive oil, garlic, salt, and black pepper. Add broccoli, tomatoes, and watercress. Toss to blend. Serve immediately.

Turkey Meat Loaf

I love comfort food. And it's even better when you boost the color, fiber, taste, and nutrition, like the AICR does with this unique recipe.

SERVES 5.

Ingredients

1/2 pound ground turkey breast

1/2 pound ground turkey

1/3 cup ketchup

1 cup unseasoned whole-wheat breadcrumbs

3/4 cup onion, finely chopped

1 teaspoon dried basil

2 teaspoons dried oregano

2 cloves garlic, minced

1 large egg

1/2 cup carrots, shredded

1/4 cup fresh parsley, chopped

1/4 cup green bell pepper, minced

1/4 cup red bell pepper, minced

salt and freshly ground black pepper to taste

3 tablespoons ketchup (optional, to use as a topping)

Procedure

Preheat oven to 350°F. Combine all ingredients except 3 tablespoons of ketchup in a large bowl. Transfer mixture to a 9-x-5-inch nonstick loaf pan. Bake 1 hour, uncovered.

Remove from oven. Spread the 3 tablespoons ketchup on top, if desired. Cover lightly with foil and let meat loaf rest 10 minutes. Cut into slices and serve.

The preceding four recipes are reprinted with permission from the American Institute for Cancer Research.

MONTEL'S SNACKS

Skip the doughnuts, muffins, pastries, scones, and Danish.

These snacks are healthier—and more filling!

Trail Mix

In a sandwich-sized Baggie, combine your favorite dried fruits, raw nuts, and seeds. Some ideas are: goji berries, cashews, walnuts, pistachios, cacao beans, raisins, dried apples, dried pears, pumpkin seeds, sunflower seeds (shelled), dried mango, dried papaya.

Just make sure your dried fruit is the unsweetened variety. Some dried fruits may be packaged with a load of unnecessary sugar.

Here's a quick and easy trail mix:

Montel's Traveling Trail Mix

MAKES 4 SERVINGS.

Ingredients

$\frac{1}{4}$ cup shelled sunflower seeds

$\frac{1}{4}$ cup raw cashews

$\frac{1}{4}$ cup raisins

$\frac{1}{4}$ cup goji berries

Raw Vegetables Dipped in Hummus

Cut up your favorite veggies, such as carrots, broccoli, and tomatoes, and dip them in this healthy hummus.

Traditional Hummus

Ingredients

2 cups canned garbanzo beans, drained

$\frac{1}{3}$ cup sesame tahini

$\frac{1}{4}$ cup lemon juice

$\frac{1}{4}$ teaspoon salt

1–3 cloves garlic, minced

2 tablespoons olive oil

$\frac{1}{8}$–1 teaspoon cayenne pepper

1 pinch black pepper

Procedure

Process ingredients in a food processor until smooth.

Soy-Flavored Almonds

MAKES 16 SERVINGS.

Ingredients

    1 pound raw unsalted almonds with skins intact
    2 tablespoons soy sauce

Procedure

Preheat oven to 325°F. Lay out almonds on a cookie sheet and bake for 12–15 minutes, turning sheet once to ensure even baking. Carefully transfer hot almonds into a large mixing bowl and pour soy sauce onto them. Stir almonds until well coated. Spread out onto cookie sheet and allow to air dry for 45–60 minutes.

Other Snack Suggestions

Fresh Fruits: apples, bananas, pears, and oranges are all great on the go.

Water: sometimes when we feel hungry we may actually be thirsty; try a tall glass of water first.

Dried figs

THE LIVING WELL CODE

7 Simple Steps
to Supercharge Your Health
and Be Physically Reborn

1. Base your diet on a foundation of a rich variety of many different vegetables and fruits—especially in their fresh, natural, and whole states.
2. Include healthy carbohydrates from whole grains, and healthy fats and protein from foods like fish, beans, and nuts.
3. Minimize saturated and trans fats, sodium, processed foods, added sugars, and cholesterol in your diet.
4. Be mindful of your calories in and calories out, to work toward a healthy body weight.
5. Don't skip meals, deprive yourself, or go on fad diets.
6. Get regular physical activity, at least thirty to sixty minutes of moderate exercise on most days of the week.
7. Combine these steps and you can reduce your risk of many major diseases, such as:
   • cardiovascular disease
   • obesity
   • several forms of cancer
   • diabetes (type 2)
   • other diseases, including Alzheimer's disease, osteoarthritis, and macular degeneration

Note: If you eat meat and poultry, make them lean, and trim off visible fat. If you enjoy dairy products, make them nonfat or low-fat.

Acknowledgments

I thank the people who helped make this book possible, including my coauthor William Doyle, manager Melanie McLaughlin, editor Tracy Bernstein, and agent Mel Berger at William Morris.

I also thank the doctors, scientists, researchers, dietitians, and others who helped with interviews, research, and other assistance, including Walter Willett, Barbara Rolls, David Grotto, Karen Collins, Robert Eckel, James Dillard, Ralph Sacco, James Hill, Laurence Sperling, Michael Thun, Adam Kaplin, Maria Carrillo, Ann Albright, Kathrynne Holden, Alberto Ascherio, Noel Rose, Patience White, David Ludwig, Carla Wolper, Wendy Traskos, Michael Okun, Nathan Yungerberg, Didier Garcia, Arnold Nelson, Duane Knudson, Chris Freytag, Barry Beedle, Julie Gilchrist, Ian Shrier, Scott Bryan, Rachel Morgan, Barbara deLateur, Evan Gottfried, Carolyn Woodberry, Ron Prior, Niles Frantz, John Swartzberg, Lilli Link, and Larry Steinman.

Living Well Resources

Montel's Top Ten Picks for Books on Diet, Nutrition, and Fitness:

American Heart Association® No-Fad Diet: A Personal Plan for Healthy Weight Loss by the American Heart Association.

The Volumetrics Eating Plan: Techniques and Recipes for Feeling Full on Fewer Calories by Barbara Rolls.

Eat, Drink, and Be Healthy: The Harvard Medical School Guide to Healthy Eating by Walter Willett, M.D., and P. J. Skerrett.

What to Eat by Marion Nestle.

Dieting for Dummies by Jane Kirby, R.D., and the American Dietetic Association.

You: On A Diet: The Owner's Manual for Waist Management by Mehmet C. Oz, M.D., and Michael F. Roizen, M.D.

The Portion Teller Plan: The No-Diet Reality Guide to Eating, Cheating, and Losing Weight Permanently by Lisa Young, Ph.D., R.D.

Mayo Clinic Healthy Weight for Everybody by Donald Hensrud (ed.) and the Mayo Clinic.

The Mayo Clinic Plan: 10 Steps to a Healthier Life for EveryBody! by the Mayo Clinic.

The No Sweat Exercise Plan (Harvard Medical School Guide) by Harvey Simon, M.D.

Health, Nutrition, Diet, and Exercise Information

Adult BMI and Calorie Calculator:
www.bcm.edu/cnrc/caloriesneed.htm

America on the Move, a national nonprofit organization promoting active living and healthy living, funded partly by the food and beverage industry:
www.americaonthemove.org

American Cancer Society:
www.cancer.org

American College of Sports Medicine:
www.acsm.org

American Council on Exercise:
www.acefitness.org

American Diabetes Association:
diabetes.org

American Dietetic Association:
www.eatright.org

American Dietetic Association nutrition tips:
www.eatright.org/cps/rde/xchg/ada/hs.xsl/home_4602_ENU_HTML
.htm

American Heart Association:
www.americanheart.org

American Heart Association No-Fad Diet:
www.americanheart.org/presenter.jhtml?identifier=3031890

American Institute for Cancer Research:
www.aicr.org

American Parkinson's Disease Association:
www.apdaparkinson.org

Alzheimer's Association:
www.alz.org/

Alzheimer's Association, Maintain Your Brain campaign, including fitness and nutrition tips:
www.alz.org/we_can_help_brain_health_maintain_your_brain.asp

Arthritis Foundation:
www.arthritis.org

Body Mass Index (BMI) calculator, U.S. Centers for Disease Control and
Prevention:
www.cdc.gov/nccdphp/dnpa/bmi/calc-bmi.htm

Centers for Disease Control and Prevention resources on fruits and veggies:
www.fruitsandveggiesmatter.gov

Centers for Disease Control and Prevention resources on physical activity: www.cdc.gov/nccdphp/dnpa/physical/index.htm

The DASH Diet:
www.nhlbi.nih.gov/health/public/heart/hbp/dash/how_plan.html

Free sixty-four-page online book, *DASH Eating Plan*:
www.nhlbi.nih.gov/health/public/heart/hbp/dash/new_dash.pdf

FDA on mercury in fish:
www.cfsan.fda.gov/~dms/admehg3.html

Harvard School of Public Health Food Pyramids:
www.hsph.harvard.edu/nutritionsource/pyramids.html

Institute of Medicine Dietary Reference Intakes:
www.nap.edu/catalog.php?record_id=10490#toc

Montel Williams MS Foundation:
www.montelms.org

National Farmers Market Directory:
www.ams.usda.gov/farmersmarkets/map.htm

National Heart, Lung and Blood Institute resources on heart disease and obesity:
www.nhlbi.nih.gov/health/public/heart/index.htm#chol

National Institutes of Health on weight loss and dieting:
health.nih.gov/result.asp/725/29

National Parkinson Foundation:
www.parkinson.org

National Weight Control Registry:
www.nwcr.ws/

Nutrition and Physical Activity Guidelines for Cancer Prevention:
caonline.amcancersoc.org/cgi/content/full/56/5/254

Nutrition and Physical Activity During and After Cancer Treatment:
caonline.amcancersoc.org/cgi/content/full/53/5/268

Nutrition Facts labels:
www.cfsan.fda.gov/~dms/foodlab.html

Parkinson's Disease Foundation:
www.pdf.org

Parkinson's Disease: Nutrition Matters brochure:
www.npfocc.org/pdfs/nutritionmatters.pdf

Partnership for Prescription Assistance (PPA):
www.pparx.org
PPA's toll-free phone number: 1-888-4PPA-NOW

Portion distortion:
www.mypyramid.gov/steps/howmuchshouldyoueat.html

PubMed, a free government database for searching peer-reviewed medical and scientific journals:
www.pubmed.gov

University of California–Berkeley 13 Keys to a Healthy Diet:
www.wellnessletter.com/html/fw/fwNut01HealthyDiet.html

U.S. Dietary Guidelines for Americans
www.health.gov/dietaryguidelines/dga2005/recommendations.htm;
www.health.gov/dietaryguidelines/dga2005/report/HTML/A_Exec-Summary.htm

U.S. Dietary Guidelines for Americans and MyPyramid
www.health.gov/dietaryguidelines/dga2005/document/
www.mypyramid.gov

U.S. government food and nutrition information:
www.nutrition.gov

U.S. government's health-related information links:
www.consumer.gov/health.htm

U.S. government information on food safety:
www.foodsafety.gov/;
www.cfsan.fda.gov/

U.S. government information on keeping food safe to eat:
www.fsis.usda.gov/Food_Safety_Education/Food_Safety_Education_Programs/index.asp

Weight-control Information Network (WIN):
www.win.niddk.nih.gov

Weight Loss and Nutrition Myths:
win.niddk.nih.gov/publications/myths.htm

Whole Grains Council:
www.wholegrainscouncil.org

World Health Organization Report:
"Diet, Nutrition and the Prevention of Chronic Diseases":
www.fao.org/docrep/005/AC911E/AC911E00.HTM

Fruit and Vegetable Safety

Nutrition Action Healthletter, December 2006, "Fear of Fresh: How to Avoid Foodborne Illness from Fruits & Vegetables":
www.cspinet.org/nah/12_06/fearoffresh.pdf

Safe Handling of Raw Produce and Fresh-Squeezed Fruit and Vegetable Juices:
www.cfsan.fda.gov/~dms/prodsafe.html

"Shoppers Guide to Pesticides in Produce":
www.foodnews.org/pdf/EWG_pesticide.pdf;
www.foodnews.org/index.php

Fish Safety

Blue Ocean Guide to Ocean-Friendly Seafood:
www.blueocean.org/seafood/

Print out a mini-guide for your pocket or purse:
www.blueocean.org/pdfs/miniguide_color.pdf

Monterey Bay Aquarium Seafood Guide:
www.mbayaq.org/cr/seafoodwatch.asp

Print out a pocket guide:
www.mbayaq.org/cr/cr_seafoodwatch/download.asp

Oceans Alive Best and Worst Seafood Choices:
www.oceansalive.org/eat.cfm?subnav=bestandworst

Print out a chart for your pocket or purse:
www.environmentaldefense.org/documents/1980_pocket_seafood_se-
lector.pdf

U.S. Department of Health and Human Services and Environmental
Protection Agency resources:
www.cfsan.fda.gov/~frf/sea-mehg.html;
www.cfsan.fda.gov/~dms/admehg3.html;
www.epa.gov/ost/fish;
www.fda.gov/bbs/topics/news/2004/NEW01038.html

Healthy Recipes

American Institute for Cancer Research:
www.aicr.org/site/PageServer?pagename=dc_rc_home

Fruit and Veggie Nutritional Databases:
www.fruitsandveggiesmorematters.org/?page_id=115 vvv

Heart Healthy Home Cooking African-American Style:
www.nhlbi.nih.gov/health/public/heart/other/chdblack/cooking.htm

Heart Healthy Latino Recipes:
www.nhlbi.nih.gov/health/public/heart/other/sp_recip.htm

Produce for Better Health Foundation:
www.fruitsandveggiesmorematters.org;
www.pbhfoundation.org

Source Notes

p. 17: "I am open to lots of things": *The Larry King Show,* CNN, March 6, 2006.

p. 20: Study suggested raw-foods-only diet can increase risk factors for heart disease: C. Koebnick, A. Garcia, P. Dagnelie, C. Strassner, J. Lindemans, N. Katz, C. Leitzmann, I. Hoffmann; "Long-Term Consumption of a Raw Food Diet Is Associated with Favorable Serum LDL Cholesterol and Triglycerides but also with Elevated Plasma Homocysteine and Low Serum HDL Cholesterol in Humans," *The Journal of Nutrition,* October 2005.

p. 33: *People* magazine reported on a girl in Arkansas: Richard Jerome, "Childhood Obesity: The Fight Against Fat," *People,* February 12, 2007.

p. 33: "Obesity is the terror within": Deborah Hastings, "Obesity Finds Niche in American Marketing," Associated Press Newswires, April 17, 2006.

p. 35: 2005 study on children's TV ads: Kevin Freking, "Children's Ads Show Lots of Junk," Associated Press Newswires, March 28, 2007.

p. 35–36: Romano's Macaroni Grill sodium information: Romano's Macaroni Grill Web site, 2007 update.

p. 39: UCLA "Diets Don't Work" study and quotes: T. Mann, A. Tomiyama, E. Westling, A. Lew, B. Samuels, J. Chatman; "Medicare's Search for Effective Obesity Treatments: Diets Are Not the Answer," *American Psychologist*, April 2007; Michael Bott, "Dieting Does Not Work, University of California, Los Angeles Researchers Report," *US Federal News*, April 3, 2007; "UC-Davis: Diets Do Not Work, UCLA Researchers Say," The California Aggie Via U-Wire, April 26, 2007; Fiona Macrae, Michelle Cazzulino, "The Horrible Truth That We Have All Suspected: Diets Just Make You Fat," *Daily Telegraph* (UK), April 11, 2007.

p. 42: The Living Well Code: discussions of evidence that healthy eating, regular physical activity, and healthy body weight can reduce the risks of cardiovascular disease, obesity, several forms of cancer, and type 2 diabetes: see for example, U.S Dietary Guidelines for Americans, 2005 (http://www.health.gov/dietaryguidelines/dga2005/recommendations.htm); World Health Organization report: "Diet, Nutrition, and the Prevention of Chronic Diseases," 2003 (http://www.fao.org/docrep/005/AC911E/AC911E00.HTM); and Walter Willett and Patrick J. Skerrett, *Eat, Drink, and Be Healthy: The Harvard Medical School Guide to Healthy Eating* (New York: Free Press, 2005), passim.

Discussions of evidence that healthy eating, regular physical activity, and healthy body weight can reduce the risks of Alzheimer's disease: see interview in this book with Maria Carrillo, director of medical and scientific relations for the Alzheimer's Association. Also see: N. Scarmeas, Y. Stern, M. Tang, R. Mayeux, J. Luchsinger, "Mediterranean Diet and Risk for Alzheimer's Disease," *Annals of Neurology*, June 2006; S. Pope, V. Shue, C. Beck, "Will a Healthy Lifestyle Help Prevent Alzheimer's Disease?", *Annual Review of Public Health*, January 2003; and M. Weih, J. Wiltfang and J. Kornhuber, "Nonpharmacologic Prevention of Alzheimer's Disease: Nutritional and Lifestyle Risk Factors," *Journal of Neural Transmission*, September 2007.

Discussions of evidence that healthy eating, regular physical activity and healthy body weight can reduce the risks of osteoarthritis: see interview in this book with Dr. Patience White, chief public health officer of the Arthritis Foundation. Also see Y. Wang, A. Hodge, A. Wluka, D. English, G. Giles, R. O'Sullivan, A. Forbes, F. Cicuttini, "Effect of Antioxidants on Knee Cartilage and Bone in Healthy, Middle-aged Subjects: A Cross-sectional Study," *Arthritis Research and Therapy*, July 2007; E. Roddy, M. Doherty, "Changing Lifestyles and Osteoarthritis: What Is the Evidence?", *Best Practice & Research Clinical Rheumatology*, February 2006; and W. Rejeski, B. Focht, S. Messier, T. Morgan, M. Pahor, B. Penninx, "Obese, Older Adults with Knee Osteoarthritis: Weight Loss, Exercise, and Quality of Life," *Health Psychology*, September 2002.

Discussions of evidence that healthy eating can reduce the risks of macular degeneration and cataracts: see Age-Related Eye Disease Study Research Group, "The Relationship of Dietary Carotenoid and Vitamin A, E, and C Intake with Age-Related Macular Degeneration in a Case-Control Study: AREDS Report No. 22," *Archives of Ophthalmology*, September 2007; W. Christen, S. Liu, D. Schaumberg, J. Buring, "Fruit and Vegetable Intake and the Risk of Cataract in Women," *American Journal of Clinical Nutrition*, June 2005; S. Moeller, A. Taylor, K. Tucker, M. McCullough, L. Chylack, S. Hankinson, W. Willett, P. Jacques, "Overall Adherence to the Dietary Guidelines for Americans Is Associated with Reduced Prevalence of Early Age-related Nuclear Lens Opacities in Women," *Journal of Nutrition*, July 2004; E. Cho, J. Seddon, B. Rosner, W. Willett, S. Hankinson; "Prospective Study of Intake of Fruits, Vegetables, Vitamins, and Carotenoids and Risk of Age-Related Maculopathy," *Archives of Ophthalmology*, June 2004; R. Maddox, S. Maddox, "SOS—Saving Our Sight," *US Pharmacist*, December 2004; and Willett, *Eat, Drink and Be Healthy*, pages 139, 180, 181. Note: Recent studies have focused on possible protective effects against macular degeneration by vitamin C and zinc, and two pigments, lutein and zeaxanthin, that are often found in dark green leafy vegetables.

p. 45: "Eat food. Not too Much": Michael Pollan, "Unhappy Meals," *New York Times Magazine*, January 28, 2007.

p. 50: For discussions of evidence of possible connections between diet, physical activity, and sexual function, see: E. Selvin, A. Burnett, E. Platz, "Prevalence and Risk Factors for Erectile Dysfunction in the U.S.," *American Journal of Medicine,* February 2007; C. Saigal, H. Wessells, J. Pace, M. Schonlau, T. Wilt, "Predictors and Prevalence of Erectile Dysfunction in a Racially Diverse Population," *Archives of Internal Medicine,* January 2006; K. Esposito et al., "Dietary Factors in Erectile Dysfunction," "Mediterranean Diet Improves Erectile Function in Subjects with the Metabolic Syndrome," *International Journal of Impotence Research,* July 2006; K. Esposito et al., "Mediterranean Diet Improves Sexual Function in Women with the Metabolic Syndrome," *International Journal of Impotence Research,* September 2007; K. Esposito et al., "Obesity, the Metabolic Syndrome, and Sexual Dysfunction," *International Journal of Impotence Research,* September 2005; K. Esposito et al., "Sexual Dysfunction and the Mediterranean Diet," *Public Health Nutrition,* December 2006.

p. 53: "Disease prevention might not be attributable": Lyn Steffen, "Eat Your Fruit and Vegetables," *Lancet,* January 28, 2006.

p. 98: Study of seventeen thousand Americans and "salad, salad dressing, and raw vegetable consumption": L. Su, L. Arab, "Salad and Raw Vegetable Consumption and Nutritional Status in the Adult US Population: Results from the Third National Health and Nutrition Examination Survey," *Journal of the American Dietetic Association,* September 2006.

p. 98: Study suggesting fat helps the body absorb nutrients: Tara Parker-Pope, "Fat Helps You Absorb Vegetables' Nutrients," *The Wall Street Journal,* August 13, 2006.

p. 98: Salads help with weight control, study by Professor Barbara Rolls: B. Rolls, L. Roe, J. Meengs; "Salad and Satiety: Energy Density and Portion Size of a First-course Salad Affect Energy Intake at Lunch," *Journal of the American Dietetic Association*, October 2004.

p. 106: World Health Organization on fish consumption: *Population Nutrient Intake Goals for Preventing Diet-related Chronic Diseases*, WHO, 2002.

p. 124: "there is now evidence that the Mediterranean diet benefits": A. Trichopoulou, D. Corella, M. Martínez-González, F. Soriguer, J. Ordovas, "The Mediterranean Diet and Cardiovascular Epidemiology," *Nutrition Reviews*, October 2006.

p. 143: "It's not low fat vs. low carb": Dean Ornish, "The Atkins Ornish South Beach Zone Diet," *Time*, June 21, 2004.

p. 143: "If you're trying to lose weight": Walter Willett and Mollie Katzen, *Eat, Drink, and Weigh Less* (New York: Hyperion, 2006), p. 12.

p. 143: "The laws of physics govern weight loss": Julian Kesner, "The Top 20 Diet Myths," *New York Daily News*, January 2, 2007.

p. 146: "A combination of regular exercise": aicr.org Web site, consulted 2007.

p. 146: "Maintaining a healthy weight isn't about going on a diet": "Say No to Yo-yo!", *OK Magazine*, August 7, 2007.

pp. 161–62: American College of Sports Medicine and the American Heart Association tips: W. Haskell, I. Lee, R. Pate, K. Powell, S. Blair, B. Franklin, C. Macera, G. Heath, P. Thompson, A. Bauman; "Recommendation for Adults from the American College of Sports Medicine and the American Heart Association," *Circulation*, August 2007.

p. 165: "Walking may be as close to a magic bullet": Regina Nuzzo, "Walking: No Pain, Results in Plenty of Gain," *Vancouver Sun*, March 29, 2007.

p. 166: Study of thirteen thousand people on walking: "A Walk a Day" fact sheet, American Council on Exercise Web site, 2007.

p. 167: Calories burned by walking: R.J. Ignelzi, "Fitness Walking," *The San Diego Union-Tribune*, October 31, 2006.

p. 205: Too much salt killing 145,000 Americans every year: Bonnie Liebman, "The Scoop on Salt," *Nutrition Action Healthletter*, July 1, 2005.

p. 206: AMA call to revoke salt's status: Sally Squires, "Rx for Salt: Cut It Out," *The Washington Post*, June 20, 2006.

p. 207: "Just one cup of canned soup": "AMA Calls for Measures to Reduce Sodium Intake in U.S. Diet; Urges FDA to Revoke 'Generally Recognized As Safe' Status," press release via U.S. Newswire, June 13, 2006.

p. 207: "There is no nutritional benefit to sea salts": Jenny Hope, "There's Not a Grain of Truth in Sea Salt Being Better for Your Health," *Daily Mail*, October 4, 2005.

p. 209: "Lowering sodium can reduce the risk": Linda Antinoro, "New Shake-up over Sodium Aims to Reduce High Blood Pressure," *Environmental Nutrition*, January 1, 2007.

p. 225: "no nutritional agent has to date been shown": Hubert Fernandez, Ramon Rodriguez, Frank Skidmore, Michael Okun, *A Practical*

Approach to Movement Disorders: Diagnosis and Surgical and Medical Management (New York: Demos Medical Publishing, 2007), p. 264.

p. 249–50: "A healthy breakfast has been shown": R.J. Ignelzi, "Running on Empty," *The San Diego Union-Tribune*, June 13, 2006.

p. 253: "We ought to think of soft drinks as a treat": Bonnie Liebman, "Morning Star," *Nutrition Action Healthletter*, January 1, 2007.

p. 255: Study and quotes by UCLA researchers on "convenience" foods: Tara Parker-Pope, "The Myth of Convenience," *The Wall Street Journal*, August 7, 2007; and "Convenience Foods Save Little Time for Working Families at Dinner," UCLA Press Release, August 7, 2007.

About the Authors

MONTEL WILLIAMS is an Emmy Award–winning talk-show host, a decorated former naval intelligence officer, an entrepreneur, motivational speaker, and philanthropist.

He is the author of the *New York Times* bestselling inspirational memoirs *Climbing Higher* and *Mountain, Get Out of My Way*, and the coauthor of the *New York Times* bestseller *BodyChange*.

Prior to hosting his own television show, Montel was a special-duty intelligence officer in the navy, specializing in cryptology. A graduate of the Naval Academy, he received a number of military awards and citations during his naval career. Before attending the Academy, he enlisted in the Marine Corps after graduating from a Baltimore, Maryland–area high school.

In 2005 he was named chairman of the National Veterans Association (NVA) and has taped public-service announcements for both the NVA and the Paralyzed Veterans of America (PVA).

Montel has worked with an array of charitable organizations, including the Make-A-Wish Foundation, the Joey DiPaolo AIDS Foundation, Diamonds for Humanity, and the Humane Society of the United States. Currently, he serves on the boards of the We Are Family Foundation, devoted to promoting tolerance and diversity through educational programs aimed at the youth of America; the PVA; and the Montel Williams MS Foundation.

In 1999, Montel announced his diagnosis with MS, a potentially debilitating autoimmune disease that affects the brain and spinal cord. To raise both awareness and funds for MS research, he created the Montel Williams MS Foundation.

In 2006 Montel became National Spokesperson for the Partnership for Prescription Assistance, a major industry campaign to extend prescription drug help to all Americans.

WILLIAM DOYLE is an award-winning writer based in New York. Once clinically obese, he lost nearly forty pounds and has kept it off for years by following the basic principles in this book.

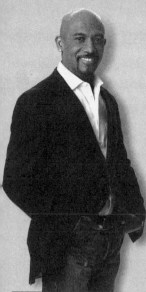
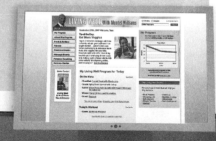